Violence

Editor

JAMES L. KNOLL IV

PSYCHIATRIC CLINICS OF NORTH AMERICA

www.psych.theclinics.com

December 2016 • Volume 39 • Number 4

ELSEVIER

1600 John F. Kennedy Boulevard • Suite 1800 • Philadelphia, Pennsylvania, 19103-2899

http://www.theclinics.com

PSYCHIATRIC CLINICS OF NORTH AMERICA Volume 39, Number 4
December 2016 ISSN 0193-953X, ISBN-13: 978-0-323-47750-5

Editor: Lauren Boyle
Developmental Editor: Kristen Helm

Psychiatric Clinics of North America (ISSN 0193-953X) is published quarterly by Elsevier Inc., 360 Park Avenue South, New York, NY 10010-1710. Months of issue are March, June, September, and December. Business and Editorial Offices: 1600 John F. Kennedy Blvd., Suite 1800, Philadelphia, PA 19103-2899. Periodicals postage paid at New York, NY and additional mailing offices. Subscription prices are $300.00 per year (US individuals), $598.00 per year (US institutions), $100.00 per year (US students/residents), $365.00 per year (Canadian individuals), $455.00 per year (international individuals), $753.00 per year (Canadian & international institutions), and $220.00 per year (Canadian & international students/residents). Foreign air speed delivery is included in all *Clinics'* subscription prices. All prices are subject to change without notice. **POSTMASTER:** Send address changes to *Psychiatric Clinics of North America*, Elsevier Health Sciences Division, Subscription Customer Service, 3251 Riverport Lane, Maryland Heights, MO 63043. **Customer Service: 1-800-654-2452 (US). From outside the United States, call 1-314-447-8871. Fax: 1-314-447-8029. E-mail: journalscustomerservice-usa@elsevier.com (for print support) and journalsonline support-usa@elsevier.com (for online support).**

Reprints. For copies of 100 or more, of articles in this publication, please contact the Commercial Reprints Department, Elsevier Inc., 360 Park Avenue South, New York, New York 10010-1710. Tel.: 212-633-3874, Fax: 212-633-3820, E-mail: reprints@elsevier.com.

Psychiatric Clinics of North America is covered in *MEDLINE/PubMed (Index Medicus), Current Contents/Social and Behavioral Sciences, Social Science Citation Index, Embase/Excerpta Medica,* and PsycINFO.

Contributors

EDITOR

JAMES L. KNOLL IV, MD
Director of Forensic Psychiatry; Professor, Division of Forensic Psychiatry, SUNY Upstate Medical University, Syracuse, New York

AUTHORS

LISA ANACKER, MD
Resident, Department of Psychiatry, University of Michigan, Ann Arbor, Michigan

BRAD D. BOOTH, MD, FRCPC
Integrated Forensic Program, Royal Ottawa Mental Health Care Group; Assistant Professor, Department of Psychiatry, University of Ottawa, Ottawa, Ontario, Canada

MICHAEL A. CUMMINGS, MD
California Department of State Hospitals (DSH), Psychopharmacology Resource Network, DSH-Patton, Patton, California

KAYLA FISHER, MD, JD
Patton State Hospital, California Department of State Hospitals, Patton, California; Department of Psychiatry, University of California, Riverside School of Medicine, Riverside, California

SUSAN HATTERS FRIEDMAN, MD
Associate Professor, Department of Psychological Medicine, University of Auckland, Grafton, Auckland, New Zealand

JACQUELINE GENZMAN, BA
Department of Psychology, University of Nebraska-Lincoln, Lincoln, Nebraska

RYAN HALL, MD
Assistant Professor, Department of Psychiatry, University of Central Florida College of Medicine; Affiliate Assistant Professor, University of South Florida; Adjunct Faculty Member, Barry University Dwayne O. Andreas School of Law, Lake Mary, Florida

NOLAN P. HUGHES, MD
Assistant Professor of Psychiatry; Associate Medical Director of Psychiatric Emergency Services, Western Psychiatric Institute and Clinic, Pittsburgh, Pennsylvania

DREW A. KINGSTON, PhD
Integrated Forensic Program, Royal Ottawa Health Care Group, Brockville Mental Health Centre (BMHC), Brockville; Departments of Psychology and Psychiatry, University of Ottawa, Ottawa, Ontario, Canada

JAMES L. KNOLL IV, MD
Director of Forensic Psychiatry; Professor, Division of Forensic Psychiatry, SUNY Upstate Medical University, Syracuse, New York

MIRANDA McEWAN, PhD
Department of Psychological Medicine, University of Auckland, Auckland, New Zealand

J. REID MELOY, PhD
Faculty, San Diego Psychoanalytic Center; Clinical Professor of Psychiatry, University of California, San Diego, La Jolla, California

JONATHAN M. MEYER, MD
California Department of State Hospitals (DSH), Psychopharmacology Resource Network, DSH-Patton, Patton, California; Department of Psychiatry, University of California, San Diego, La Jolla, California

DOUGLAS MISQUITTA, MD
Assistant Professor, Department of Psychiatry and Behavioral Health, Ohio State University Wexner Medical Center, Columbus, Ohio

BRITTA OSTERMEYER, MD, MBA
The Paul and Ruth Jonas Chair; Professor; Chairman, Department of Psychiatry and Behavioral Sciences, University of Oklahoma, Oklahoma City, Oklahoma

DEBRA A. PINALS, MD
Director, Program in Psychiatry, Law and Ethics; Clinical Professor, Department of Psychiatry, University of Michigan, Ann Arbor, Michigan

GEORGE PROCTOR, MD
California Department of State Hospitals (DSH), Psychopharmacology Resource Network, DSH-Patton, Patton, California

JOHN S. ROZEL, MD
Assistant Professor of Psychiatry; Medical Director of re:solve Crisis Network, Western Psychiatric Institute and Clinic, Pittsburgh, Pennsylvania

PHILIP SARAGOZA, MD
Adjunct Clinical Assistant Professor of Psychiatry, University of Michigan Medical School, Ann Arbor, Michigan

DELANEY SMITH, MD
Associated Faculty; Clinical Assistant Professor, Department of Psychiatry and Behavioral Health, Ohio State University Wexner Medical Center; Twin Valley Behavioral Healthcare, Columbus, Ohio

RILEY SMITH, MD
Assistant Clinical Professor of Physical Medicine and Rehabilitation, Wayne State University/Beaumont, Dearborn, Michigan

RENEE SORRENTINO, MD
Instructor, Department of Psychiatry, Harvard School of Medicine, Boston, Massachusetts

STEPHEN M. STAHL, MD, PhD
Director of Psychopharmacology Services, California Department of State Hospitals (DSH), Sacramento, California; Department of Psychiatry, University of California, San Diego, La Jolla, California

KEITH R. STOWELL, MD
Assistant Professor of Psychiatry; Medical Director of Psychiatric Emergency Services, Western Psychiatric Institute and Clinic, Pittsburgh, Pennsylvania

STEPHEN G. WHITE, PhD
President, Work Trauma Services, Inc, San Francisco, California; Associate Clinical Professor, Department of Psychiatry, University of California at San Francisco, Lafayette, California

BG (Ret) STEPHEN N. XENAKIS, MD, US Army
Former Erik Erikson Scholar, The Austen Riggs Center, Stockbridge, Massachusetts

Contents

> Persistent violence not due to acute psychosis or mania can be managed only after appropriate characterization of the aggressive episodes (psychotic, impulsive, or predatory/planned/instrumental). The type of violence combined with the psychiatric diagnosis dictates the evidence-based pharmacologic approaches for psychotically motivated and impulsive aggression, whereas instrumental violence mandates forensic/behavioral strategies. For nonacute inpatients, schizophrenia spectrum disorders, traumatic brain injury, and dementia comprise the majority of individuals who are persistently aggressive, with impulsive actions being the most common form of violence across all diagnoses. Neurobiological considerations combined with empirical data provide a comprehensive framework for systematic medication trials to manage persistently aggressive patients.

> Violence is common in the emergency department (ED). The ED setting has numerous environmental risk factors for violence, including poor staffing, lack of privacy, overcrowding, and ready availability of nonsecured equipment that can be used as weapons. Strategies can be taken to mitigate the risk of violence toward health care workers, including staff training, changes to the ED layout, appropriate use of security, and policy-level changes. Health care providers in the ED should be familiar with local case law and standards related to the duty to warn third parties when a violent threat is made by a patient.

> Inpatient violence constitutes a major concern for staff, patients, and administrators. Violence can cause physical injury and psychological trauma. Although violence presents a challenge to inpatient clinicians, it should not be viewed as inevitable. By looking at history of violence, in addition to clinical and other historical factors, clinicians can identify which patients present the most risk of exhibiting violent behavior and whether the violence would most likely flow from psychosis, impulsivity, or predatory characteristics. With that information, clinicians can provide environmental and treatment modifications to lessen the likelihood of violence.

of conducting violent operations, and the psychology of violence fundamentally anchors its professionalism. The occurrence of unwanted violence and tragic incidence of suicides, homicides, and abuse expose the challenges to containing the behavior outside of the combat and training theaters.

PSYCHIATRIC CLINICS OF NORTH AMERICA

FORTHCOMING ISSUES

March 2017
Clinical Issues and Affirmative Treatment with Transgender Clients
Lynne Carroll and Lauren Mizock, *Editors*

June 2017
Women's Mental Health
Susan G. Kornstein and Anita H. Clayton, *Editors*

September 2017
Behavioral Emergencies
Nidal Moukaddam and
Veronica Theresa Tucci, *Editors*

RECENT ISSUES

September 2016
Adverse Effects of Psychotropic Treatments
Rajnish Mago, *Editor*

June 2016
Schizophrenia: Advances and Current Management
Peter F. Buckley, *Editor*

March 2016
Bipolar Depression
John L. Beyer, *Editor*

RELATED INTEREST

Child and Adolescent Psychiatric Clinics of North America, April 2014 (Vol. 23, No. 2)
Disaster and Trauma
Stephen J. Cozza, Judith A. Cohen, and Joseph G. Dougherty, *Editors*
Available at: http://www.childpsych.theclinics.com/

THE CLINICS ARE AVAILABLE ONLINE!
Access your subscription at:
www.theclinics.com

Preface

The Study of Violence: An Act of Species Consciousness

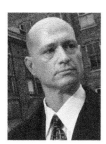

James L. Knoll IV, MD
Editor

Why did they kill little Bobby Franks? Not for money, not for spite; not for hate. They killed him as they might kill a spider or a fly, for the experience. They killed him because they were made that way.
— *Clarence Darrow (Leopold & Loeb trial)[1]*

When Nathan Leopold and Richard Loeb kidnapped and murdered 14-year-old Robert Franks in 1924, it was described as the "crime of the century."[2] The trial became a media spectacle, and the greatest legal and forensic minds of the time were involved. Sigmund Freud, suffering from cancer, was offered any price he asked by William Randolph Hearst to come to the United States to "psychoanalyze" Leopold and Loeb. Freud prudently declined, citing the fact that he had not personally evaluated the defendants.

Part of the reason the Leopold and Loeb trial captured international attention was that the two were privileged and intelligent—yet sought to commit the "perfect crime." Surely this was a natural experiment in the psychology of violence. Nature and nurture could, ostensibly, be removed from the equation. Both came from impressive lineages. Leopold was a child prodigy who had a genius IQ, spoke five languages, and was raised by a wealthy family. Loeb was the son of a wealthy lawyer and vice president of Sears, Roebuck, & Company. He skipped several grades and became the youngest person to graduate from the University of Michigan at age 17. To this day, their motive is debated: existential "thrill kill" versus mere greed.

Almost 80 years later, I encountered a similar scenario. As medical director of psychiatric services for the New Hampshire state prison system, I witnessed the prison's reception of Parker and Tulloch—2001's redux of Leopold and Loeb.[3] Parker and Tulloch were relatively privileged teens who killed an innocent couple—two beloved Dartmouth professors. Parker and Tulloch saw themselves as smarter than the average

Psychiatr Clin N Am 39 (2016) xiii–xiv
http://dx.doi.org/10.1016/j.psc.2016.08.001
0193-953X/16/© 2016 Published by Elsevier Inc.

psych.theclinics.com

person and planned to take money from the professors to furnish a new, adventurous life in Australia. I had become a forensic psychiatrist out of an interest to understand violent criminal behavior. Like many before me, I found that working in corrections and the criminal justice system provided an abundance of tragic sadness to counterbalance the violent aggression. Yet, in truth, this was apparent to me from an early age.

When I was a boy of about 10 years old, I happened upon a *TIME* magazine cover displaying a large vat of Kool-Aid surrounded by some 900 dead bodies. The image stuck with me. When an elementary school teacher gave my class the assignment of writing a short story, I wrote a piece from the perspective of a Jonestown member who managed to escape by feigning death. I can only speculate on my teacher's reaction to my work. In hindsight, I suspect this was an early warning sign I might become a forensic psychiatrist. Decades later, I interviewed and lectured with a few of the only living survivors of the Jonestown Tragedy. Having come full circle, it was apparent to me that tragedy and violence are intertwined, eternal companions.[4]

It is my contention that violence (and therefore tragedy) calls on us to take a more substantive, meaningful look at how we hope to transcend this instinctual challenge as a species. It is a call to face ourselves with an open and fearless heart. In the final analysis, regardless of "what social or biological factors are involved, ultimately we must take responsibility for our anger."[5] The scholarly articles on violence in this issue of the *Psychiatric Clinics of North America* are a step in this direction. I am grateful to all my colleagues for their thoughtful work and contributions to this issue—all have long ago accepted the challenge to face the problem of violence with a fearless heart. It is my hope that readers will appreciate this and carry forward the work of harm reduction with an eye toward "species consciousness"—our sense of shared fate and undeniable interconnectedness.[6] It is no less a matter than our survival and progress.

James L. Knoll IV, MD
Division of Forensic Psychiatry
SUNY Upstate Medical University
600 East Genesee Street, Suite 108
Syracuse, NY 13202, USA

E-mail address:
knollj@upstate.edu

REFERENCES

1. Weinberg A, Douglas JWO. Attorney for the damned: Clarence Darrow in the courtroom; Reprint edition. Chicago: University of Chicago Press; 2012.
2. Higdon H. Leopold and Loeb: the crime of the century. Champaign (IL): University of Illinois Press; 1999.
3. Lehr D, Zuckoff M. Judgment Ridge: the true story behind the Dartmouth murders. New York: HarperCollins; 2003.
4. Knoll J. Afterword. In: Kaczynski D, editor. Every Last Tie: The Story of the Unabomber and His Family. Durham (NC): Duke University Press Books; 2016.
5. Leifer R. Vinegar into honey. Ithaca (NY): Snow Lion Press; 2008.
6. Lifton RJ. Witness to an extreme century: a memoir. New York: Free Press; 2011.

Psychopharmacology of Persistent Violence and Aggression

Jonathan M. Meyer, MD[a,b,*], Michael A. Cummings, MD[a],
George Proctor, MD[a], Stephen M. Stahl, MD, PhD[b,c]

KEYWORDS

- Aggression • Violence • Impulsivity • Pharmacology

KEY POINTS

- Impulsive behavior is the most common form of persistent aggression among psychiatric inpatients. Psychotic and impulsive violence are amenable to pharmacotherapy. Predatory behavior demands forensic/behavioral approaches.

- For schizophrenia patients, D_2 antagonism with plasma-level monitoring is the initial strategy. Clozapine has strong evidence for treating psychotic aggression in refractory patients and for impulsive violence. The evidence for adjunctive strategies to antipsychotics is weak for psychotic and impulsive violence.

- The traumatic brain injury (TBI) literature contains only a small number of good-quality randomized clinical trials (RCTs) that demonstrate efficacy in persistent aggression: centrally acting β-blockers, divalproex, or carbamazepine and possibly dopaminergic agonists. There is no literature to support the use of antipsychotics.

- Evidence-based pharmacotherapy for persistently aggressive dementia patients includes use of acetylcholinesterase inhibitors (AChEIs) for mild–moderate stage patients and selective serotonin reuptake inhibitors (SSRIs). Antipsychotics carry dose-dependent mortality risks. The data for valproate also show increased risk for mortality risk and poor tolerability.

Disclosures: Dr M.A. Cummings and Proctor report no disclosures. Dr J.M Meyer reports having received speaking or advising fees from Alkermes, Forum, Merck, Otsuka-USA, and Sunovion. Dr S.M. Stahl reports having received advising fees, consulting fees, speaking fees, and/or research grants from Acadia, Alkermes, Biomarin, Clintara, Eli-Lilly, EnVivo, Forest, Forum, GenoMind, JayMac, Lundbeck, Merck, Novartis, Orexigen, Otsuka-USA, PamLabs, Pfizer, RCT Logic, Servier, Shire, Sprout, Sunovion, Sunovion-UK, Taisho, Takeda, Teva, Tonix, and Trius.

[a] California Department of State Hospitals (DSH), Psychopharmacology Resource Network, DSH-Patton, 3102 East Highland Avenue, Patton, CA 92369, USA; [b] Department of Psychiatry, University of California, San Diego; 9500 Gilman Drive, MC 0603, La Jolla, CA 92093-0603, USA; [c] California Department of State Hospitals (DSH), Bateson Building, 1600 9th Street, Room 400, Sacramento, CA 95814, USA
* Corresponding author.
E-mail address: jmmeyer@ucsd.edu

Psychiatr Clin N Am 39 (2016) 541–556
http://dx.doi.org/10.1016/j.psc.2016.07.012
0193-953X/16/© 2016 Elsevier Inc. All rights reserved.

psych.theclinics.com

INTRODUCTION

Violence and aggression are major societal concerns and often intersect with psychiatric providers in both acute and subacute settings.[1] Although the terms, *aggression* and *violence*, are often used synonymously, there are distinct differences in their meanings. Aggression represents acts that may lead to harm (toward self or others), whereas violence is a subcategory of aggressive acts that causes harm to others.[2] The presentation of aggression in unmedicated or inadequately treated psychiatric patients is often dramatic and associated with agitation, yet these patients often respond robustly in the short term to standard pharmacologic interventions, including antipsychotics alone or with benzodiazepines.[1,3–5] (For a comprehensive review, see Newman.[2]) The more vexing clinical issue is the management of persistent aggression toward others encountered in psychiatric inpatient and forensic settings.[6] Although the diagnostic mix in these environments weighs heavily toward schizophrenia spectrum diagnoses, intellectual disability, and cognitive disorders, clinicians must accurately classify the nature of aggressive events before embarking on any pharmacologic course of action. Such categorization is critical to the determination of appropriate management strategies that are necessarily based on the interplay between underlying psychiatric diagnosis and the nature of the violent episodes.[7]

The purpose of this review is to provide a rational therapeutic approach to the problem of persistent aggression and violence seen in long-term psychiatric inpatient settings and focus on how the categorization of violent acts informs medication strategies within the most common diagnostic groups: schizophrenia spectrum disorders, TBI, and dementia. Self-injurious behavior and other aggressive acts toward self, as well as the acute management of agitation in minimally treated patients, are not discussed to focus attention on the more intractably aggressive patient. The treatment of behavioral disturbance in nonpsychotic patients with intellectual disabilities is typically confined to specialized facilities designed to meet the unique needs of this population. Readers are referred to several excellent reviews for discussions about the appropriateness and nature of pharmacotherapy for aggressive patients with intellectual disabilities.[8–11]

Although pharmacologic approaches may be useful, and necessary, for certain types of violence, it must be noted that environmental variables, staffing ratios and expertise, and psychosocial stressors play an important role in aggressive behavior. These areas must also be addressed to obtain the maximum benefit from medication options.[6]

Classification of Aggression

Although persistent violence has long been recognized among chronic psychiatric inpatients, only in the past decade has there emerged a clinically useful and empirically derived categorization scheme. Investigators within the New York State Hospital system videotaped a series of assaults and then supplemented the videos with assailant and victim interviews to determine the motivation for each violent act.[12] These detailed assessments led the investigators to conclude that 3 categories could be used to define these aggressive acts: psychotic, impulsive, and predatory (also called organized or instrumental). Despite that a majority of patients had schizophrenia spectrum diagnoses, the investigators were intentionally agnostic regarding the underlying psychopathology, thereby acknowledging that a patient with schizophrenia might engage in violence for psychotic reasons (due to delusions and hallucinations), as an impulsive overreaction to a perceived threat, or for purely manipulative purposes. This research also clarified that impulsive violence is the most common form seen among chronic psychiatric inpatients, despite the high prevalence of psychosis. This finding, and the construct validity of the 3-factor approach, was confirmed by subsequent research within the California state hospital system. After reviewing records on 839 assaults committed by 88 persistently aggressive patients with schizophrenia as the modal diagnosis, the most common type of assault was impulsive (54%), followed by organized (29%) and psychotic (17%) (**Table 1**).[13] These empirically derived data have also informed the science of risk prediction. The third-generation of violence risk assessment instruments (eg, Historical Clinical Risk Management-20, Version 3) was an improvement over older unstructured or actuarial methods and uses a structured professional judgment approach based on static historical elements, dynamic factors, and the type of aggressive acts.[14] These newer risk assessment tools better define the appropriate clinical interventions to reduce aggression by incorporating a more complex picture of the aggressive individual and the context for violence.[14]

Neurobiology of Persistent Impulsive Aggression

The pharmacologic treatment of psychotically motivated aggression initially follows a well-defined path from D_2 antagonism to clozapine, followed by adjunctive strategies, whereas that for organized violence requires behavioral techniques and/or custodial approaches.[6] The pharmacologic approach to impulsive violence is much more heterogeneous and depends greatly on the neurobiological substrate as reflected by the primary diagnosis and the failure of medication regimens.[15–17] Although threat response is mediated by a circuit that encompasses periaqueductal gray matter, hippocampus, amygdala, and hypothalamus, it is the prefrontal cortex (PFC) that determines the nature of the threat and the response.[18] PFC dysfunction thereby increases the risk of impulsive aggressive responses by failing to make appropriate risk/reward assessments for inhibiting aggressive responses. Thus, ventromedial PFC lesions increase impulsive aggression "not because the aggressive response is disinhibited, but rather because the costs and benefits of engaging in impulsive aggression are not properly represented."[18]

Although the connections between the ventromedial PFC and amygdala serve a top-down inhibitory function, there are positive bottom-up processes from the amygdala to orbital PFC structures whose dysfunction may play a role in the conversion of impulsive actions to more compulsive behaviors.[16] There is also in vivo and human evidence for the role of the insula in addictions and other compulsive behavior.[19]

Table 1
Proportion of inpatient aggressive acts by subtypes

Psychotic (17%)	Predatory/Organized (29%)	Impulsive (54%)
• Behavior motivated by positive symptoms of psychosis (hallucinations, delusions)	• Planned behavior with clear goals in mind (eg, intimidation, retribution, monetary or material gain) • Behavior not obviously a response to threat or provocation • Often accompanied by limited autonomic arousal	• Behavior precipitated by provocation, threat, stress • Often associated with fear, anger, frustration • High levels of autonomic arousal

From Stahl SM. Deconstructing violence as a medical syndrome: mapping psychotic, impulsive, and predatory subtypes to malfunctioning brain circuits. CNS Spectrums 2014;19:358; with permission.

Conceptually, the persistently aggressive patient with impulsivity can be viewed as someone whose bottom-up processes have reinforced the behavior to the extent that it has become compulsive.

Several pharmacologic strategies for treating persistent aggression are suggested by data correlating dysfunction in serotonin and dopamine systems associated with PFC-amygdala connectivity. Increased rates of impulsive aggression in animal and human studies are associated with findings consistent with serotonergic hypofunction, including increased serotonin 2A receptor availability in the orbital PFC,[17] tryptophan depletion studies,[20] and polymorphisms of the serotonin transporter and monoamine oxidase A genes that are associated with lower synaptic serotonin availability.[21] Decreased PFC dopaminergic signaling is also associated with aggression,[20] especially with polymorphisms in more than one gene regulating dopamine turnover.[22] There is difficulty in applying many of these findings to psychiatric inpatients due to the monoaminergic dysfunction inherent in illnesses, such as schizophrenia[23]; however, certain insights can be applied as part of a systematic approach toward managing the persistently aggressive inpatient. The ensuing discussion focuses on the pharmacologic management of psychotic and impulsive aggression within common diagnostic inpatient categories, because the evidence is most robust for these forms of aggression. Although patients may engage in multiple forms of aggression, organized or instrumental violence is generally not amenable to pharmacotherapy.

Schizophrenia

Psychotic violence and aggression

Psychotic violence and aggression are the direct products of poorly controlled positive symptoms of psychosis; therefore, their treatment is consistent with known algorithms for managing inadequate responders.[6,24,25] Patients with a diagnosis of schizoaffective disorder, bipolar type, may not respond sufficiently to antipsychotic monotherapy, and mood stabilization is often necessary to control partially remitted mania or hypomania that continues to drive psychotic symptoms.[26] Retrospective analyses of large outpatient schizophrenia trials in Europe and the United States have drawn inferences about the antiaggression effects of antipsychotics based on improvement in the Positive and Negative Syndrome Scale (PANSS) hostility item[27,28]; however, whether such findings translate into efficacy differences among persistently violent inpatients is unknown. Even among prospective studies of aggressive schizophrenia patients, the failure to distinguish among predatory, impulsive, or psychotic violence limits the applicability of the data to those with psychotically motivated acts.[29]

Once an act of violence has been characterized as psychotically motivated aggression, the pharmacologic approach is consistent with that for the management of treatment-resistant schizophrenia. In persistently violent schizophrenia patients not exhibiting neurologic adverse effects from treatment (eg, extrapyramidal symptoms, and akathisia), plasma antipsychotic levels are critical to determining whether lack of expected medication response is due to insufficient D_2 antagonism for kinetic or adherence reasons or is due to pharmacodynamic failure (eg, treatment refractoriness) despite plasma levels at the upper limit of tolerability (**Table 2**).[30] The determination of whether low plasma antipsychotic levels represent an adherence issue or a pharmacokinetic one requires an understanding of each agent's metabolic pathways, and the expected concentration:dose relationships in patients who are extensive metabolizers and not receiving enzyme inhibitors or inducers. **Table 3** presents data for commonly used agents in long-term inpatient settings. Because ultrarapid metabolizer phenotypes exist for cytochrome P450 2D6, and to a lesser extent for

Table 2
Selected antipsychotic response and tolerability thresholds

Drug	Response Threshold	Tolerability Threshold	Plasma Level Associated with 80% D_2 Antagonism
Haloperidol	3–5 ng/mL[84]	20 ng/mL[84]	2.0 ng/mL[85]
Fluphenazine	0.81 ng/mL[84]	3.0 ng/mL[84]	Unknown (2.23 ng/mL = 89% occupancy)[86]
Olanzapine	21 ng/mL[87]	176 ng/mL[88]	73 ng/mL[89]
Risperidone + 9-OH Risperidone (active moiety)	20 ng/mL[90]	Poorly defined	45 ng/mL[91]

Table 3
Antipsychotic Concentration/Oral Dose (C/D) Relationships

Drug	Relationships and Supporting Data
Aripiprazole	Concentration (ng/mL) = 12 × oral dose (mg/d) Aripiprazole/Dehydroaripiprazole Ratio: 4.4 (range 3.6–5.0)[92] Aripiprazole Dehydroaripiprazole[92] 10 mg/d → 126 ± 78 ng/mL 35 ± 4 ng/mL 20 mg/d → 230 ± 193 ng/mL 46 ± 37 ng/mL 30 mg/d → 400 ± 236 ng/mL 83 ± 18 ng/mL
Clozapine	• 40 year old male, 80 kg, clozapine/norclozapine ratio of 1.32 Concentration (ng/mL) = 1.08 × oral dose (mg/d) (nonsmokers) Concentration (ng/mL) = 0.67 × oral dose (mg/d) (smokers) 325 mg → 350 ng/mL[93] (nonsmokers) 525 mg → 350 ng/mL[93] (smokers) • 40 year old female, 70 kg, clozapine/norclozapine ratio of 1.32 Concentration (ng/mL) = 1.32 × oral dose (mg/d) (nonsmokers) Concentration (ng/mL) = 0.80 × oral dose (mg/d) (smokers) 265 mg → 350 ng/mL[93] (nonsmokers) 435 mg → 350 ng/mL[93] (smokers)
Haloperidol	Concentration (ng/mL) = 0.78 × oral dose (mg/d) 2 mg/d → 1.57 ± 1.42 ng/mL[94] 10 mg/d → 7.79 ± 4.79 ng/mL[95]
Fluphenazine	Concentration (ng/mL) = 0.08 × oral dose (mg/d) (nonsmokers) Concentration (ng/mL) = 0.04 × oral dose (mg/d) (smokers) 22.9 mg → 1.83 ± 0.94 ng/mL[96] (nonsmokers) 20.4 mg → 0.89 ± 0.43 ng/mL[96] (smokers)
Olanzapine	Concentration (ng/mL) = 2.00 × oral dose (mg/d) (nonsmokers) Concentration (ng/mL) = 1.43 × oral dose (mg/d) (smokers) 10 mg → 20 ng/mL[97] (nonsmokers) 14 mg → 20 ng/mL[98] (smokers)
Risperidone + 9-OH Risperidone (active moiety)	Active Moiety Concentration (ng/mL) = 7.00 × oral dose (mg/d) Risp/9-OH Risp Ratio: 0.2 (range 0.1–0.3)[99] 2 mg/d → C/D Ratio = 7.05[100] 6 mg/d → C/D Ratio = 7.15[100] 10 mg/d → C/D Ratio = 7.28[100] 16 mg/d → C/D Ratio = 6.95[100]

cytochrome P450, genetic testing should only be considered for persistently low plasma levels once the possibility of poor adherence has been addressed (eg, switching to a long-acting injectable formulation). The development of extrapyramidal symptoms or akathisia signals the termination of any antipsychotic trial, with clozapine the next logical step; however, there is a small proportion of patients who do not experience neurologic adverse effects even at high dosages and plasma concentrations,[31] stressing the value of plasma antipsychotic levels to ascertain whether a point of futility has been reached.[30]

Clozapine remains the antipsychotic of choice for treatment refractory schizophrenia, with response rates averaging 50% to 60%.[32] In double-blind schizophrenia trials with strict definitions of treatment refractoriness using Kane criteria, response rates to olanzapine, even at high doses are usually less than 10%.[33] Trough plasma-level monitoring is exceedingly useful for optimizing clozapine therapy, because response rates are low for levels less than 350 ng/mL.[34] Clinicians should be familiar with the management of clozapine's adverse effects, because it represents the only evidence-based option for treatment of refractory schizophrenia.[35] Adjunctive medications (eg, anticonvulsants, lithium, and antidepressants) and antipsychotic combinations have limited evidence for the treatment of refractory psychosis,[36] with the exception of potent D_2 antagonists or aripiprazole added to clozapine.[36]

Impulsive violence and aggression

Among state hospital patients, impulsive violence is the most common form of aggression.[13] In these patients, clozapine also emerges as the preferred agent, and its antiaggressive property in these individuals is independent of its impact on psychotic symptoms. Evidence for this assertion comes from studies, such as that by Krakowski and colleagues,[37] who performed a randomized, double-blind, parallel-group, 12-week trial in physically assaultive New York State Hospital patients with schizophrenia or schizoaffective disorder. The mean baseline PANSS total score for this group was 85, and the study patients were 80% male with mean age 34, mean illness duration 15 years, and an average of 11 prior psychiatric hospitalizations. Subjects were randomly assigned to treatment with clozapine (n = 37), olanzapine (n = 37), or haloperidol (n = 36), and both the number and severity of all aggressive events were measured by the Modified Overt Aggression Scale (MOAS). At study end there were nonsignificant numeric changes in PANSS total scores across all groups, but clozapine significantly reduced MOAS verbal, physical, and total aggression scores compared with haloperidol or olanzapine.[37] Clozapine's effect was more pronounced in those with cognitive dysfunction, despite that poor executive function at study baseline predicted higher levels of aggression.[38] Further evidence that clozapine's antiaggression effect is independent of its antipsychotic properties can also be seen in the literature,[39] including a small case series of clozapine therapy for impulsive aggression among nonpsychotic patients with antisocial personality disorders.[40] Not only did clozapine significantly decrease rates of impulsive aggression and violence in this cohort but also it did so at serum levels below 350 ng/mL, with level mean 171 ng/mL.

The evidence for adjunctive strategies to clozapine is surprisingly weak and consists primarily of case series and open-label studies. When there is an insufficient response to clozapine despite maximization of plasma clozapine levels and augmentation of clozapine with more potent D_2 antagonism, the evidence-based options for persistent aggression in schizophrenia patients include valproate, centrally acting β-adrenergic antagonists, and SSRI antidepressants.[41,42] Lithium has compelling evidence for antiaggressive effects,[43] but the data in schizophrenia patients are limited.[44] If lithium or valproate is used, it should be used at high therapeutic serum levels with appropriate safety monitoring and should be withdrawn after 8 weeks unless there is compelling evidence of response in order avoid the additive weight gain seen when combined with antipsychotic therapy. As a method of improving PFC top-down control over behavior, clinicians at a California state hospital described a series of 5 clozapine-treated schizophrenia spectrum patients with persistent impulsive aggression who responded to adjunctive extended-release methylphenidate (Concerta).[45] There was a significant reduction in aggressive events to the extent that one frequently aggressive patient became eligible for discharge. Moreover, there was no evidence that methylphenidate exacerbated underlying psychotic symptoms, even at daily doses up to 72 mg.

Traumatic Brain Injury

Nonpsychotic patients with TBI often require psychiatric intervention and at times hospitalization specifically to manage persistent impulsive violence and aggression. A broad array of agents has been tried in this population, including older and newer antipsychotics, anticonvulsants, lithium, antidepressants (primarily SSRIs), psychostimulants, and drugs that modulate noradrenergic neurotransmission (eg, β-adrenergic antagonists and α_2-adrenergic agonists).[46] Although there are anecdotal reports of success for many of these agents, systematic reviews are much less positive in their assessment of efficacy.[3,46] A 2016 review by a panel of French experts concluded, "There is insufficient evidence to standardize drug treatments for these disorders." Although the literature in this area is comprised primarily of low-quality data, with few studies meeting criteria for level IB evidence (derived from at least 1 randomized controlled trial [RCT]) or even level IIA evidence (derived from at least 1 controlled study without randomization), there are data to suggest that certain medications can be used in a manner consistent with good clinical practice.

A 2009 Cochrane review noted that the published literature to date included only 6 RCTs of medications for TBI-related aggression, of which 4 evaluated β-blockers (propranolol and pindolol), with 1 study each for methylphenidate and the weak dopamine agonist amantadine. Based on this small number of RCTs, only the centrally acting β-blockers (eg, propranolol) had strong evidence for efficacy.[3] Although antipsychotics are often used to manage aggression in the TBI population, detailed reviews of individual atypical antipsychotic agents shows an absence of level IIa or level Ib data, and evidence that antipsychotics may be associated with significant cognitive, neurologic, and other adverse effects.[47] The 2016 French article reached similar conclusions in stating bluntly, "There is no evidence of efficacy for neuroleptics."[46]

Aside from β-blockers, there was sufficient accrued data since the 2009 Cochrane meta-analysis for the French group to state that carbamazepine and valproate seem effective for agitation and aggression and are recommended as first line treatment. Between these 2 anticonvulsants, carbamazepine has several disadvantages, including the need for slow titration to minimize ataxia and sedation, risk of hyponatremia, and potent induction of both cytochrome P450 3A4 and the efflux transporter P-glycoprotein that may result in a clinically significant reduction in serum levels of other medications.[48,49] Certain Asian patients commencing carbamazepine treatment must also be screened for the HLA-B*1502 allele due its association with carbamazepine-induced Stevens-Johnson syndrome.[50] Valproic acid preparations (eg, divalproex) are not without their clinical limitations, as noted in **Table 4**, but divalproex has a lower incidence of gastrointestinal side effects than does valproic acid (ie, Depakene) and can be loaded up to 30 mg/kg in 24 hours.[51] Lithium has shown positive results for aggression in open-label studies of patients with intermittent explosive

Table 4
Divalproex and carbamazepine comparison

	Forms	Baseline Labs	Clinical Issues	Therapeutic Level
Carbamazepine	• Tablet • Chewable Tablet • Extended-release tablet • Suspension	• Complete blood cell count • Serum sodium • HLA-B1502 in certain Asian groups • Consider plasma/serum levels of medications with expected pharmacokinetic interactions	• Cannot be loaded • Pharmacokinetic interactions with numerous medications • Hyponatremia	6.0–12.0 µg/mL
Divalproex (valproate)	• Tablet • Sprinkles • Extended-release tablet • Syrup	• Complete blood cell count • Liver function tests • Consider plasma/serum levels of medications with expected pharmacokinetic interactions	• Weight gain • Tremor • Hyperammonemia • Thrombocytopenia	60–120 µg/mL

disorder,[44] but there are insufficient data to recommend this for TBI-related violence. Antidepressants, in particular SSRIs, do show efficacy for depressive symptoms in TBI patients but not for aggression and violence.[46]

The appeal of dopaminergic agonists for persistently violent TBI patients rests within the same theoretic construct as its use in impulsively violent schizophrenia patients with inadequate response to clozapine. Although methylphenidate would be expected to produce a more robust effect on PFC control of impulsive behavior than weaker dopamine agonists, such as amantadine, there are no good-quality RCTs for methylphenidate in TBI patients.[52] One double-blind RCT of amantadine, 100 mg twice daily, versus placebo in 76 irritable or aggressive TBI patients more than 6 months postinjury showed positive results,[53] but a subsequent study with the same amantadine dose in a larger cohort (n = 168) did not show statistically significant between-group differences in observer ratings at day 28 or at day 60.[54]

Dementia

The dementia population consists of a heterogeneous group of disorders, but a majority of studies have focused on the most common cause, Alzheimer disease (AD), and to a lesser extent on vascular dementia. As with TBI, numerous classes of medications have been tried to treat persistent aggression in this population, and practice has evolved due to the morbidity and mortality concerns surrounding certain psychotropics.[55,56] Important to the assessment of agitation in dementia patients is consideration of physical limitations due to uncorrected visual and hearing impairments, environmental issues (eg, poor lighting) and physical symptoms, such as pain.[57] The routine use of nonopioid analgesics, at times empirically due to a patient's limited verbal abilities, must be considered, especially if violence episodes are centered around the provision of care or other physical manipulations.[57] Behavioral interventions ranging from exercise to music to bright light therapy have some positive studies, although it should be noted that the efficacy data for psychosocial interventions is modest, often due to methodological issues with study design.[57–59] Nonetheless, these interventions do not carry the safety concerns seen with certain psychotropics.

Among pharmacologic options for persistent aggression in dementia patients, the strongest evidence points to the benefits of AChEIs for neuropsychiatric symptoms of mild to moderate AD.[60,61] Studies have noted differential response to specific AChEIs, so inadequate response to 1 agent does not preclude the trial of another.[61,62] Memantine has also shown evidence of efficacy both as monotherapy[61] and when combined with AChEIs.[62] When starting AChEIs, the recommended titration should be followed to decrease the risk of diarrhea and other gastrointestinal complaints. These agents should only be used after consultation with a cardiologist in patients with decreased sinus node automaticity or atrioventricular block due to vagotonic effects on sinoatrial and atrioventricular nodes.[63] In memantine clinical trials, the only adverse effect seen in greater than or equal to 5% of patients and at least twice the incidence of placebo was headache (6% vs 3%) and for the extended-release formulation dizziness (5% vs 1%).[64]

In addition to the AChEIs, the other medication class with significant positive results in aggressive dementia patients is the SSRI antidepressants. A 2011 Cochrane review noted the small number of controlled studies at that time, yet concluded that the SSRIs sertraline and citalopram reduced symptoms of agitation compared to placebo (2 trials), and also stated that SSRIs and trazodone seemed to be reasonably well tolerated compared with placebo and to antipsychotics.[65] A subsequent double-blind, placebo-controlled 9-week trial of citalopram, 30 mg/d, in 186 AD patients with clinically significant agitation found that citalopram was effective and was associated with a reduction in delusions (odds ratio = 0.40), anxiety (odds ratio = 0.43), and irritability/lability (odds ratio = 0.38).[66] A secondary analysis indicated that those who experienced greater response tended to have certain baseline features — outpatients, those with moderate agitation, and those with lower levels of cognitive impairment — whereas patients with more severe agitation and greater cognitive impairment tended to experience more adverse effects.[67] Study participation itself had a significant impact on the outcome, with significant response also seen in the placebo cohort, a finding that may underestimate the true treatment effect of citalopram outside of a clinical trial.[68] Because QTc warnings exist for citalopram and escitalopram,[69] sertraline is an alternative SSRI, especially in a patient population more prone to cardiac events.[65] Trazodone is typically started at doses no higher than 12.5 mg or 25 mg to assess orthostasis risk. Over time, low-dose trazodone can be used multiple times per day, with patients tolerating doses up to 200 mg/d with careful titration.[70]

Atypical antipsychotics were investigated extensively for the neuropsychiatric complications in AD, but safety concerns arose with respect to cerebrovascular adverse effects and increased mortality rates.[71,72] Although meta-analyses did find that certain agents could reduce psychosis and aggression, in large double-blind studies there was no separation from placebo.[73] Moreover, the mortality signal for antipsychotics seen in early randomized controlled studies,[71] was seen in large naturalistic data sets, such as that from the US Veterans Health Administration (VHA) (n = 46,008).[56,74] After controlling for numerous demographic, medical, and psychiatric diagnostic factors, in the 180 days after starting an antipsychotic, the absolute mortality risk difference among veterans with dementia ranged from 3.2% to 12.3%

across all antipsychotics, whereas antidepressant exposure decreased mortality risk.[56] The number needed to harm for mortality from antipsychotics ranged from 8 for haloperidol to 31 for quetiapine. The risk:benefit equation has thus tilted away from routine use of antipsychotics in persistently aggressive dementia patients unless other behavioral approaches and other treatment alternatives have been explored and proved ineffective.[57–59]

When compelled to use an antipsychotic, typical agents, such as haloperidol, should be avoided due to higher mortality and neurologic adverse event rates. Very low doses of risperidone (starting at 0.25 mg at bedtime and rarely exceeding 1.0 mg/d due to risk of falls)[75] or quetiapine (starting at 25 mg twice a day and rarely exceeding 150 mg/d) can be considered.[76] Efforts should be made to taper off these agents over time as studies have shown that a significant proportion of dementia patients can be successfully weaned from antipsychotics without behavioral deterioration.[77]

Although anticonvulsants show efficacy in violent TBI patients, the accrued evidence in dementia patients is largely negative, aside from small case series and open-label studies. Multiple RCTs for valproate (or divalproex) have shown no efficacy, leading to the conclusion that valproate in any form should not be used routinely for aggression related to dementia.[78,79] The data for carbamazepine are conflicting, and both tolerability and kinetic concerns limit its use.[78] In the large VHA retrospective study, valproate exposure was also analyzed and was found associated with an increased mortality risk difference of 5.1%, which translates to an number needed to harm of 20.[56] Although valproate monotherapy has exhibited limited benefit, if there is clinical efficacy for valproate in dementia patients, it may possibly be seen when combined with other agents, and at relatively low serum levels (40–60 μg/mL).[80] Nonetheless, even at low serum levels, valproate may be poorly tolerated. Data with other anticonvulsants are confined to small open-label studies, but one 16-week trial in 40 inpatients showed modest benefit from low-dose lamotrigine (mean dose at study endpoint 46.3 ± 24.4 mg/d, range 25–100 mg/d) to the extent that the doses of concomitant antipsychotics could be lowered.[81] Although benzodiazepines are occasionally used on an emergent basis for acute agitation, there is no evidence to support their efficacy for persistent aggression or violence, with significant concerns about tolerability.[82,83]

SUMMARY

Persistent violence presents significant challenges and safety issues within inpatient psychiatric facilities. Accurate diagnosis and familiarity with the neurobiology and categorization of the 3 types of violence can direct clinicians toward the best evidence-based combinations of treatment interventions. This categorization is critical, because medications are ineffective for organized/predatory/instrumental violence, and treatment lies primarily in the realm of environmental and psychosocial interventions. Although psychotic violence is the least common form, it is arguably the easiest to address by eliminating undertreated and treatment refractory schizophrenia through antipsychotic plasma-level monitoring and through increased clozapine use. Impulsive violence is the most prevalent form of persistent violence in schizophrenia patients, and clozapine's antiaggressive properties are also effective in these individuals. Although there are a limited number of proved strategies for violence reduction for inpatients with TBIs or dementia, it is imperative that research continues to elucidate effective treatments for these groups, as the psychiatric population changes and ages.

ACKNOWLEDGMENTS

The authors would like to recognize Laura J. Dardashti, MD; Jennifer O'Day, MD; and Eric Schwartz, MD, for their contributions to this article.

REFERENCES

1. Citrome L, Volavka J. The psychopharmacology of violence: making sensible decisions. CNS Spectr 2014;19:411–8.
2. Newman WJ. Psychopharmacologic management of aggression. Psychiatr Clin North Am 2012;35:957–72.
3. Fleminger S, Greenwood RJR, Oliver DL. Pharmacological management for agitation and aggression in people with acquired brain injury. Cochrane Database Syst Rev 2006;(4):CD003299.
4. Ballard C, Corbett A. Agitation and aggression in people with Alzheimer's disease. Curr Opin Psychiatry 2013;26:252–9.
5. Gillies D, Sampson S, Beck A, et al. Benzodiazepines for psychosis-induced aggression or agitation. Cochrane Database Syst Rev 2013;(4):CD003079.
6. Stahl SM, Morrissette DA, Cummings M, et al. California State Hospital Violence Assessment and Treatment (Cal-VAT) guidelines. CNS Spectr 2014;19:449–65.
7. Szabo KA, White CL, Cummings SE, et al. Inpatient aggression in community hospitals. CNS Spectr 2015;20:223–30.
8. Sabaawi M, Singh NN, de Leon J. Guidelines for the use of clozapine in individuals with developmental disabilities. Res Dev Disabil 2006;27:309–36.
9. de Leon J, Greenlee B, Barber J, et al. Practical guidelines for the use of new generation antipsychotic drugs (except clozapine) in adult individuals with intellectual disabilities. Res Dev Disabil 2009;30:613–69.
10. Tsiouris JA. Pharmacotherapy for aggressive behaviours in persons with intellectual disabilities: treatment or mistreatment? J Intellect Disabil Res 2010;54: 1–16.
11. de Leon J, editor. A Practitioner's guide to prescribing antiepileptics and mood stabilizers for adults with intellectual disabilities. New York: Springer Science + Business Media, LLC; 2012.
12. Nolan KA, Czobor P, Roy BB, et al. Characteristics of assaultive behavior among psychiatric inpatients. Psychiatr Serv 2003;54:1012–6.
13. Quanbeck CD, McDermott BE, Lam J, et al. Categorization of aggressive acts committed by chronically assaultive state hospital patients. Psychiatr Serv 2007;58:521–8.
14. McDermott BE, Holoyda BJ. Assessment of aggression in inpatient settings. CNS Spectr 2014;19:425–31.
15. Siever LJ. Neurobiology of aggression and violence. Am J Psychiatry 2008;165: 429–42.
16. Stahl SM. Deconstructing violence as a medical syndrome: mapping psychotic, impulsive, and predatory subtypes to malfunctioning brain circuits. CNS Spectr 2014;19:357–65.
17. Rosell DR, Siever LJ. The neurobiology of aggression and violence. CNS Spectr 2015;20:254–79.
18. Blair RJ. The neurobiology of impulsive aggression. J Child Adolesc Psychopharmacol 2016;26:4–9.
19. Belin-Rauscent A, Daniel ML, Puaud M, et al. From impulses to maladaptive actions: the insula is a neurobiological gate for the development of compulsive behavior. Mol Psychiatry 2016;21(4):491–9.

20. Seo D, Patrick CJ, Kennealy PJ. Role of serotonin and dopamine system interactions in the neurobiology of impulsive aggression and its comorbidity with other clinical disorders. Aggress Violent Behav 2008;13:383–95.

21. Pavlov KA, Chistiakov DA, Chekhonin VP. Genetic determinants of aggression and impulsivity in humans. J Appl Genet 2012;53:61–82.

22. Grigorenko EL, De Young CG, Eastman M, et al. Aggressive behavior, related conduct problems, and variation in genes affecting dopamine turnover. Aggress Behav 2010;36:158–76.

23. Hoptman MJ. Impulsivity and aggression in schizophrenia: a neural circuitry perspective with implications for treatment. CNS Spectr 2015;20:280–6.

24. Stahl SM, Morrissette DA. Should high dose or very long-term antipsychotic monotherapy be considered before antipsychotic polypharmacy?. In: Ritsner MS, editor. Polypharmacy in psychiatry practice, Volume I: multiple medication use strategies. New York: Springer; 2013. p. 107–26.

25. Morrissette DA, Stahl SM. Treating the violent patient with psychosis or impulsivity utilizing antipsychotic polypharmacy and high-dose monotherapy. CNS Spectr 2014;19:439–48.

26. Vieta E. Developing an individualized treatment plan for patients with schizoaffective disorder: from pharmacotherapy to psychoeducation. J Clin Psychiatry 2010;71(Suppl 2):14–9.

27. Volavka J, Czobor P, Derks EM, et al. Efficacy of antipsychotic drugs against hostility in the European First-Episode Schizophrenia Trial (EUFEST). J Clin Psychiatry 2011;72:955–61.

28. Volavka J, Czobor P, Citrome L, et al. Effectiveness of antipsychotic drugs against hostility in patients with schizophrenia in the Clinical Antipsychotic Trials of Intervention Effectiveness (CATIE) study. CNS Spectr 2014;19:374–81.

29. Victoroff J, Coburn K, Reeve A, et al. Pharmacological management of persistent hostility and aggression in persons with schizophrenia spectrum disorders: a systematic review. J Neuropsychiatry Clin Neurosci 2014;26:283–312.

30. Meyer JM. A rational approach to employing high plasma levels of antipsychotics for violence associated with schizophrenia: case vignettes. CNS Spectr 2014;19:432–8.

31. Simpson GM, Kunz-Bartholini E. Relationship of individual tolerance, behavior and phenothiazine produced extrapyramidal system disturbance. Dis Nerv Syst 1968;29:269–74.

32. Citrome L. Handbook of treatment-resistant schizophrenia. London (United Kingdom): Springer Healthcare Ltd.; 2013.

33. Conley RR, Kelly DL, Richardson CM, et al. The efficacy of high-dose olanzapine versus clozapine in treatment-resistant schizophrenia: a double-blind, crossover study. J Clin Psychopharmacol 2003;23:668–71.

34. Remington G, Agid O, Foussias G, et al. Clozapine and therapeutic drug monitoring: is there sufficient evidence for an upper threshold? Psychopharmacology (Berl) 2013;225:505–18.

35. Bleakley S, Taylor D. Clozapine handbook. Warwickshire (United Kingdom): Lloyd-Reinhold Communications; 2013.

36. Taylor DM, Smith L, Gee SH, et al. Augmentation of clozapine with a second antipsychotic - a meta-analysis. Acta Psychiatr Scand 2012;125:15–24.

37. Krakowski MI, Czobor P, Citrome L, et al. Atypical antipsychotic agents in the treatment of violent patients with schizophrenia and schizoaffective disorder. Arch Gen Psychiatry 2006;63:622–9.

38. Krakowski MI, Czobor P. Executive function predicts response to antiaggression treatment in schizophrenia: a randomized controlled trial. J Clin Psychiatry 2012; 73:74–80.

39. Frogley C, Taylor D, Dickens G, et al. A systematic review of the evidence of clozapine's anti-aggressive effects. Int J Neuropsychopharmacol 2012;15: 1351–71.

40. Brown D, Larkin F, Sengupta S, et al. Clozapine: an effective treatment for seriously violent and psychopathic men with antisocial personality disorder in a UK high-security hospital. CNS Spectr 2014;19:301–402.

41. Goedhard LE, Stolker JJ, Heerdink ER, et al. Pharmacotherapy for the treatment of aggressive behavior in general adult psychiatry: a systematic review. J Clin Psychiatry 2006;67:1013–24.

42. Citrome L, Volavka J. Pharmacological management of acute and persistent aggression in forensic psychiatry settings. CNS Drugs 2011;25:1009–21.

43. Muller-Oerlinghausen B, Lewitzka U. Lithium reduces pathological aggression and suicidality: a mini-review. Neuropsychobiology 2010;62:43–9.

44. Jones RM, Arlidge J, Gillham R, et al. Efficacy of mood stabilisers in the treatment of impulsive or repetitive aggression: systematic review and meta-analysis. Br J Psychiatry 2011;198:93–8.

45. Skoretz P, Tang C. Stimulant medications for treatment of impulsive violence in schizophrenic female forensic patients: a case series. CNS Spectrums 2016. [Epub ahead of print].

46. Plantier D, Luaute J. Drugs for behavior disorders after traumatic brain injury: Systematic review and expert consensus leading to French recommendations for good practice. Ann Phys Rehabil Med 2016;59:42–57.

47. Elovic EP, Jasey NN Jr, Eisenberg ME. The use of atypical antipsychotics after traumatic brain injury. J Head Trauma Rehabil 2008;23:132–5.

48. Zaccara G, Perucca E. Interactions between antiepileptic drugs, and between antiepileptic drugs and other drugs. Epileptic Disord 2014;16:409–31.

49. Akamine Y, Uehara H, Miura M, et al. Multiple inductive effects of carbamazepine on combined therapy with paliperidone and amlodipine. J Clin Pharm Ther 2015;40:480–2.

50. Tangamornsuksan W, Chaiyakunapruk N, Somkrua R, et al. Relationship between the HLA-B*1502 allele and carbamazepine-induced Stevens-Johnson syndrome and toxic epidermal necrolysis: a systematic review and meta-analysis. JAMA Dermatol 2013;149:1025–32.

51. Miller BP, Perry W, Moutier CY, et al. Rapid oral loading of extended release divalproex in patients with acute mania. Gen Hosp Psychiatry 2005;27:218–21.

52. Sami MB, Faruqui R. The effectiveness of dopamine agonists for treatment of neuropsychiatric symptoms post brain injury and stroke. Acta Neuropsychiatr 2015;27:317–26.

53. Hammond FM, Bickett AK, Norton JH, et al. Effectiveness of amantadine hydrochloride in the reduction of chronic traumatic brain injury irritability and aggression. J Head Trauma Rehabil 2014;29:391–9.

54. Hammond FM, Sherer M, Malec JF, et al. Amantadine effect on perceptions of irritability after traumatic brain injury: results of the Amantadine Irritability Multisite Study. J Neurotrauma 2015;32:1230–8.

55. Langballe EM, Engdahl B, Nordeng H, et al. Short- and long-term mortality risk associated with the use of antipsychotics among 26,940 dementia outpatients: a population-based study. Am J Geriatr Psychiatry 2014;22(4):321–31.

56. Maust DT, Kim HM, Seyfried LS, et al. Antipsychotics, other psychotropics, and the risk of death in patients with dementia: number needed to harm. JAMA Psychiatry 2015;72:438–45.

57. McClam TD, Marano CM, Rosenberg PB, et al. Interventions for Neuropsychiatric Symptoms in Neurocognitive Impairment Due to Alzheimer's Disease: A Review of the Literature. Harv Rev Psychiatry 2015;23:377–93.

58. Ballard C, Orrell M, YongZhong S, et al. Impact of Antipsychotic Review and Nonpharmacological Intervention on Antipsychotic Use, Neuropsychiatric Symptoms, and Mortality in People With Dementia Living in Nursing Homes: A Factorial Cluster-Randomized Controlled Trial by the Well-Being and Health for People With Dementia (WHELD) Program. Am J Psychiatry 2016;173:252–62.

59. Richter T, Meyer G, Mohler R, et al. Psychosocial interventions for reducing antipsychotic medication in care home residents. Cochrane Database Syst Rev 2012;(12):CD008634.

60. Cummings J, Lai TJ, Hemrungrojn S, et al. Role of donepezil in the management of neuropsychiatric symptoms in Alzheimer's Disease and Dementia with Lewy Bodies. CNS Neurosci Ther 2016;22:159–66.

61. Cumbo E, Ligori LD. Differential effects of current specific treatments on behavioral and psychological symptoms in patients with Alzheimer's disease: a 12-month, randomized, open-label trial. J Alzheimers Dis 2014;39:477–85.

62. Gareri P, Putignano D, Castagna A, et al. Retrospective study on the benefits of combined Memantine and cholinEsterase inhibitor treatMent in AGEd Patients affected with Alzheimer's Disease: the MEMAGE study. J Alzheimers Dis 2014;41:633–40.

63. Eisai Inc. Aricept [Package Insert]. Woodcliff Lake, NJ 07677: Eisai Inc; 2015.

64. Forest Pharmaceuticals Inc. Namenda XR [Package Insert]. St Louis, MO 63045: Forest Pharmaceuticals LLC; 2014.

65. Seitz DP, Adunuri N, Gill SS, et al. Antidepressants for agitation and psychosis in dementia. Cochrane Database Syst Rev 2011;(2):CD008191.

66. Leonpacher AK, Peters ME, Drye LT, et al. Effects of Citalopram on Neuropsychiatric Symptoms in Alzheimer's Dementia: Evidence From the CitAD Study. Am J Psychiatry 2016;173(5):473–80.

67. Schneider LS, Frangakis C, Drye LT, et al. Heterogeneity of treatment response to citalopram for patients with Alzheimer's Disease with aggression or agitation: the CitAD randomized clinical trial. Am J Psychiatry 2016;173(5):465–72.

68. Rosenberg PB, Drye LT, Porsteinsson AP, et al. Change in agitation in Alzheimer's disease in the placebo arm of a nine-week controlled trial. Int Psychogeriatr 2015;27:2059–67.

69. Tampi RR, Balderas M, Carter KV, et al. Citalopram, QTc prolongation, and torsades de pointes. Psychosomatics 2015;56:36–43.

70. Teri L, Logsdon RG, Peskind E, et al. Treatment of agitation in AD: a randomized, placebo-controlled clinical trial. Neurology 2000;55:1271–8.

71. Schneider LS, Dagerman KS, Insel P. Risk of death with atypical antipsychotic drug treatment for dementia: meta-analysis of randomized placebo-controlled trials. JAMA 2005;294:1934–43.

72. Ballard C, Waite J. The effectiveness of atypical antipsychotics for the treatment of aggression and psychosis in Alzheimer's disease. Cochrane Database Syst Rev 2006;(1):CD003476.

73. Schneider LS, Tariot PN, Dagerman KS, et al. Effectiveness of atypical antipsychotic drugs in patients with Alzheimer's disease. N Engl J Med 2006;355:1525–38.

74. Kales HC, Kim HM, Zivin K, et al. Risk of mortality among individual antipsychotics in patients with dementia. Am J Psychiatry 2012;169:71–9.
75. Katz I, de Deyn PP, Mintzer J, et al. The efficacy and safety of risperidone in the treatment of psychosis of Alzheimer's disease and mixed dementia: a meta-analysis of 4 placebo-controlled clinical trials. Int J Geriatr Psychiatry 2007;22: 475–84.
76. Tariot PN, Profenno LA, Ismail MS. Efficacy of atypical antipsychotics in elderly patients with dementia. J Clin Psychiatry 2004;65(Suppl 11):11–5.
77. Declercq T, Petrovic M, Azermai M, et al. Withdrawal versus continuation of chronic antipsychotic drugs for behavioural and psychological symptoms in older people with dementia. Cochrane Database Syst Rev 2013;(3):CD007726.
78. Gallagher D, Herrmann N. Antiepileptic drugs for the treatment of agitation and aggression in dementia: do they have a place in therapy? Drugs 2014;74: 1747–55.
79. Herrmann N, Lanctot KL, Hogan DB. Pharmacological recommendations for the symptomatic treatment of dementia: the Canadian Consensus Conference on the Diagnosis and Treatment of Dementia 2012. Alzheimers Res Ther 2013;5:S5.
80. Dolder CR, Nealy KL, McKinsey J. Valproic acid in dementia: does an optimal dose exist? J Pharm Pract 2012;25:142–50.
81. Suzuki H, Gen K. Clinical efficacy of lamotrigine and changes in the dosages of concomitantly used psychotropic drugs in Alzheimer's disease with behavioural and psychological symptoms of dementia: a preliminary open-label trial. Psychogeriatrics 2015;15:32–7.
82. Bishara D, Taylor D, Howard RJ, et al. Expert opinion on the management of behavioural and psychological symptoms of dementia (BPSD) and investigation into prescribing practices in the UK. Int J Geriatr Psychiatry 2009;24:944–54.
83. Tampi RR, Tampi DJ. Efficacy and tolerability of benzodiazepines for the treatment of behavioral and psychological symptoms of dementia: a systematic review of randomized controlled trials. Am J Alzheimers Dis Other Demen 2014; 29:565–74.
84. Midha KK, Hubbard JW, Marder SR, et al. Impact of clinical pharmacokinetics on neuroleptic therapy in patients with schizophrenia. J Psychiatry Neurosci 1994;19:254–64.
85. Nyberg S, Farde L, Halldin C, et al. D2 dopamine receptor occupancy during low-dose treatment with haloperidol decanoate. Am J Psychiatry 1995;152: 173–8.
86. Nyberg S, Farde L, Halldin C. Delayed normalization of central D2 dopamine receptor availability after discontinuation of haloperidol decanoate - preliminary findings. Arch Gen Psychiatry 1997;54:953–8.
87. Perry PJ, Lund BC, Sanger T, et al. Olanzapine plasma concentrations and clinical response: acute phase results of the North American Olanzapine Trial. J Clin Psychopharmacol 2001;21:14–20.
88. Kelly DL, Richardson CM, Yu Y, et al. Plasma concentrations of high-dose olanzapine in a double-blind crossover study. Hum Psychopharmacol 2006;21: 393–8.
89. Uchida H, Takeuchi H, Graff-Guerrero A, et al. Predicting dopamine D2 receptor occupancy from plasma levels of antipsychotic drugs: a systematic review and pooled analysis. J Clin Psychopharmacol 2011;31:318–25.
90. Remington G, Mamo D, Labelle A, et al. A PET study evaluating dopamine D2 receptor occupancy for long-acting injectable risperidone. Am J Psychiatry 2006;163:396–401.

91. Gefvert O, Eriksson B, Persson P, et al. Pharmacokinetics and D2 receptor occupancy of long-acting injectable risperidone (Risperdal Consta) in patients with schizophrenia. Int J Neuropsychopharmacol 2005;8:27–36.
92. Sparshatt A, Taylor D, Patel MX, et al. A systematic review of aripiprazole–dose, plasma concentration, receptor occupancy, and response: implications for therapeutic drug monitoring. J Clin Psychiatry 2010;71:1447–556.
93. Rostami-Hodjegan A, Amin AM, Spencer EP, et al. Influence of dose, cigarette smoking, age, sex, and metabolic activity on plasma clozapine concentrations: a predictive model and nomograms to aid clozapine dose adjustment and to assess compliance in individual patients. J Clin Psychopharmacol 2004;24:70–8.
94. Kapur S, Zipursky R, Roy P, et al. The relationship between D2 receptor occupancy and plasma levels on low dose oral haloperidol: a PET study. Psychopharmacology 1997;131:148–52.
95. Wei FC, Jann MW, Lin HN, et al. A practical loading dose method for converting schizophrenic patients from oral to depot haloperidol therapy. J Clin Psychiatry 1996;57:298–302.
96. Ereshefsky L, Jann MW, Saklad SR, et al. Effects of smoking on fluphenazine clearance in psychiatric inpatients. Biol Psychiatry 1985;20:329–32.
97. Bishara D, Olofinjana O, Sparshatt A, et al. Olanzapine: a systematic review and meta-regression of the relationships between dose, plasma concentration, receptor occupancy, and response. J Clin Psychopharmacol 2013;33:329–35.
98. Haslemo T, Eikeseth PH, Tanum L, et al. The effect of variable cigarette consumption on the interaction with clozapine and olanzapine. Eur J Clin Pharmacol 2006;62:1049–53.
99. de Leon J, Wynn G, Sandson NB. The pharmacokinetics of paliperidone versus risperidone. Psychosomatics 2010;51:80–8.
100. de Leon J, Sandson NB, Cozza KL. A preliminary attempt to personalize risperidone dosing using drug–drug interactions and genetics: part II. Psychosomatics 2008;49:347–61.

Violence in the Emergency Department

Keith R. Stowell, MD*, Nolan P. Hughes, MD, John S. Rozel, MD

KEYWORDS

- Violence • Emergency psychiatry • Emergency department • Aggression
- Healthcare violence

KEY POINTS

- Violence is common in the emergency department (ED), often occurring at much higher rates than other occupations and in other health care settings.
- The ED setting has numerous environmental risk factors for violence, including poor staffing, lack of privacy, overcrowding, and ready availability of nonsecured equipment that can be used as weapons.
- Although numerous risk assessment instruments exist, they are not validated for the emergency setting and the nature of the ED environment limits their clinical utility.
- Health care providers in the ED should be familiar with local case law and standards related to the duty to warn third parties when a violent threat is made by a patient.

INTRODUCTION

The emergency department (ED) is a common site of violent presentations in health care. Individuals may present with violent ideation or threats, or after having engaged in a violent act. Additionally, violence in the ED itself is a particular concern. This article explores the prevalence of such presentations, followed by a discussion of assessment and management of violence. Related duties that arise in the care of such patients, including the duty to warn, and gun access also will be discussed.

EPIDEMIOLOGY

The Occupational Safety and Health Administration (OSHA) defines workplace violence as "any act or threat of physical violence, harassment, intimidation, or other threatening disruptive behavior that occurs at the work site." Health care workers represent one of the most at-risk groups, with rates of serious workplace incidents occurring 4 times more often in the health care setting than in private industry. OSHA indicates that the risk of serious violence against health care workers nearly matches the rate of all other industries combined.[1]

Western Psychiatric Institute and Clinic, Department of Psychiatry, University of Pittsburgh School of Medicine, 3811 Ohara Street, Pittsburgh, PA 15213, USA
* Corresponding author.
E-mail address: stowellkr@upmc.edu

Psychiatr Clin N Am 39 (2016) 557–566
http://dx.doi.org/10.1016/j.psc.2016.07.003
0193-953X/16/© 2016 Elsevier Inc. All rights reserved.

psych.theclinics.com

Within the category of health care workers, emergency room providers are among those facing the highest risk of workplace violence. The American College of Emergency Physicians (ACEP) noted that more than 75% of emergency room physicians experience at least 1 incident of workplace violence in a given year.[2] A survey of 6504 emergency room nurses found that 54.5% had experienced physical or verbal violence in the previous 7 days. Of that group, 62.2% had experienced more than 1 episode in that same 7-day period.[3] As high as these numbers are, it is quite likely that true rates are actually higher. Often, these events are viewed as being part of the job and are not properly reported. Of those identified as victims of workplace violence, 65.6% did not file a formal report for the violent event and 86.1% did not formally report verbal abuse, instead informally reporting to security, their immediate supervisor on duty, or other emergency personnel.[3] In another survey of 242 emergency room workers who were victims of workplace violence, 65% said they did not formally report the event and 64% said they had not had any violence prevention training in the preceding year.[4]

Limited data exist on the number of presentations related to violent ideation or an act of violence that preceded the ED visit. Most data in this area are related to incidence of violence occurring while in the ED.

IMPACT OF WORKPLACE VIOLENCE

The ACEP states that "protecting emergency patients and staff from violent acts is fundamental to ensuring quality patient care."[2] It is clear that violence in the emergency room is damaging beyond the event itself. In a survey of emergency nurses, 58.4% felt angry, 39.2% felt anxious, 19.2% felt frightened, and 6.4% had feelings of depression following an incident of workplace violence. More than half (57.7%) did not feel they were protected from workplace violence, and 27.2% considered leaving their job in the emergency room.[3]

A study of emergency physicians in Turkey found a significant relationship between feelings of emotional exhaustion and burnout related to exposure to violence.[5] Further, violent events have been shown to directly impact productivity and patient care. A study by Kowalenko and colleagues[6] demonstrated significant impairments in the Healthcare Productivity Survey scores for emergency workers after being victimized, including negative impacts on general productivity, ability to handle workload, and ability to handle cognitive demands, provide safe and competent care, and provide support.

ASSESSING RISK FOR VIOLENCE

Certain populations and types of emergency presentations appear to pose a higher risk of violent events while in the ED. Chief complaints that indicate mental health issues, active substance use, and acute pain portrayed higher risk of violence in the emergency room, as did being viewed as a high user of care, and entering the emergency room in police custody. A past history of violence also raises future risk, both in the emergency room and beyond.[7,8] Additional risk factors are those that are similar for other acts of violence, including male gender, younger age, criminal record, unemployment, homicidal thoughts, treatment nonadherence, unstable psychosis, impulsivity, and intellectual disability.

Factors related to the ED encounter itself may also lend themselves to an increased risk of violence. In **Box 1**, there are numerous environmental risk factors that increase the risk of violence in the ED.[9]

Box 1
Environmental risk factors that increase the risk of violence in the emergency department

Poor staffing levels

Low levels of patient-staff interaction

Lack of privacy

Overcrowding

Poor physical facilities

Availability of weapons, especially in rooms used for dual purposes (psychiatric and general medical assessment)

Adapted from Davison SE. The management of violence in general psychiatry. Adv Psychiatr Treat 2005;11:363.

ASSESSMENT TOOLS

A review by Singh and colleagues[10] identified more than 120 different risk assessment tools that had been developed to predict harmful behaviors. On narrowing the focus to the 9 most commonly used tools, Singh and colleagues[10] found that predictive validity varied widely, with tools designed to evaluate small, specific populations performing better than those attempting to be more broadly applicable. Each instrument has varying training requirements and time needed for its use. A literature review did not reveal any reliable published data on use of such instruments for specific use in the emergency room setting.

Most of the available data on use of risk assessment tools may be difficult to translate to clinical use in an emergency room. Many instruments produce a stratification of future risk, often taking the form of low, moderate, or high risk categories. Although these categories provide 1 useful component of assessment, it remains only 1 element of the clinical judgment required to determine appropriate disposition. As there are large variations in resources in a given setting, it is difficult to generalize that a certain categorical risk level requires a certain level of care. For example, someone stratified to a high risk category in a metropolitan area that has access to high-level outpatient and crisis services may be appropriately safe for discharge, when someone of the same risk category in an underserved area might not have access to similar services and thus requires hospitalization.[11] As such, the current standard of care with the emergency setting does not necessitate the use of such instruments in the ED.

DOCUMENTATION OF RISK ASSESSMENT

For patients who present with agitation, violent ideation or stated intention, or recent violent acts, completion of a risk assessment is important (**Box 2**). Documentation should include an analysis of risk factors, including those that are dynamic (modifiable) and static (unchangeable). Risk-reducing factors should also be considered and documented. Ultimately, documentation should include the risk stratification, as well as a plan that addresses mitigation of the modifiable risk factors and enhances protective factors.

SAFETY ISSUES

Managing the safety of the clinical environment requires a multimodal approach, focusing on interventions at the individual level, the physical plant, and policy level.

> **Box 2**
> **Important documentation elements in the risk assessment**
>
> Document risk-enhancing and risk-reducing factors
>
> General estimate of overall risk
>
> Analysis of risk factors
>
> Include relevant collateral data
>
> Estimate of reliability of patient and collateral informants
>
> Discuss rationale for decisions, including why a given intervention was chosen or not chosen if relevant (eg, "An involuntary commitment was considered, but not pursued because of X, Y, Z.")
>
> *Data from* Knoll JL. The psychiatric ER survival guide. Psychiatric Times. 2011. Available at: http://www.psychiatrictimes.com/risk-assessment-0/psychiatric-er-survival-guide. Accessed April 30, 2016.

Considerations include staff training, the physical layout of the ED, security, and developing guidelines on management of violent behavior and related adverse events.[12]

STAFF TRAINING

Staff training is an essential element in the prevention of violence. Such training can focus on recognizing early signs of agitation and risk factors for agitation. Deescalation techniques are particularly important areas of focus, but training in this area is often limited or nonexistent. Additional areas for training include appropriate use of medication to treat agitation, as well as the use of seclusion or restraint. Training should be provided at the outset of employment, followed by ongoing education about such issues in the form of supervision, rounds, and refresher training at certain intervals.[13]

PROJECT BETA

In 2012, the American Association for Emergency Psychiatry released Project BETA: Best Practices in the Evaluation and Treatment of Agitation. This series of articles attempted to address the inconsistency in approaches to treating agitation, which often vary widely by individual practitioner and institutional practice. Given the significant risk that agitated individuals pose in becoming aggressive and violent, a set of guidelines was developed. This series focused on 5 particular areas: medical evaluation and triage of the agitated patient, psychiatric evaluation of the agitated patient, verbal deescalation, psychopharmacologic approaches, and use and avoidance of seclusion and restraint. Of particular note in these guidelines is a discussion of the importance of verbal deescalation as being central to the overall management of agitation, often occurring concurrently with triage and initial assessment. Additional guidance is provided on the use of targeting medications toward the presumptive cause of agitation and using medications that are better tolerated and unlikely to sedate the individual to the point that psychiatric assessment can no longer occur.[14–19] These open-source journal articles are available in the *Western Journal of Emergency Medicine* and serve as helpful resources for emergency department staff: http://westjem.com/tag/volume-13-issue-1.

PHYSICAL LAYOUT AND SECURITY

The use of metal detectors in the ED has been growing. One barrier has been perceived acceptability, but findings suggest a positive perception and greater feelings of safety. Manual searches of patients and visitors arriving in the ED are also a possibility, although potentially more invasive and staff intensive. A stepped approach can be considered with an initial screening by security and removal of concerning items with subsequent manual screening if the patient is to be admitted to an inpatient unit. In addition, a ready security presence at entry and throughout the ED can be helpful for mitigating violence occurring in this setting. Additional security presence in the ED will generally lead to a quicker response time if violent acts occur in the ED.[13,20]

Box 3 contains suggestions for room adaptations and important features for security in the ED.

POLICY

At the policy level, multiple interventions ranging from involvement of organized medicine, to regulatory bodies, to local hospital practice are important. Kowalenko and colleagues[13] suggest a zero tolerance policy for violence against health care workers, as such violence is often tolerated and accepted as part of the emergency environments. Additionally, reporting of incidents is important to help drive policies and interventions aimed at reducing workplace violence. Consideration also can be given to threat alerts, which may be reviewed by hospital, departmental, and security leadership, with dissemination to staff.[13]

DUTIES TO THIRD PARTIES: UNDERSTANDING THE LEGAL AND ETHICAL PARAMETERS

When patients present with recent violent behavior or express violent ideation, issues there are potential duties that treating providers must consider. The 1976 Tarasoff decision from California was the first widely recognized legal ruling addressing potential duties of professionals to potential victims of intentional violence by their patients.

When a therapist determines, or pursuant to the standards of his profession should determine, that the patient presents a serious danger of violence to another, the therapist incurs an obligation to use reasonable care to protect the intended victim against such danger.[21]

The essential elements of the Tarasoff duty are the following:
1. A therapist-patient relationship exists
2. The therapist knows of risk by the patient against a third party

Box 3
Interview room safety issues
Easily accessible alarm systems
Unobstructed exits
Doors that open outward, cannot be locked from inside, allow easy access from the outside in event of emergency
Barrier-resistant doors, which contain a small compact door within the door
Location close to staff areas
Removal of all potential weapons, especially in multipurpose rooms
Unobstructed viewing window
Furniture layout, including heavy furniture that is secured to the ground
Adapted from Davison SE. The management of violence in general psychiatry. Adv Psychiatr Treat 2005;11:363.

3. The harm is severe or potentially life threatening
4. The risk is imminent
5. The target is known or readily identifiable

Tarasoff was only the starting point. In the ensuing 40 years, every state (including California) has since developed its own distinct application or reinterpretation of the original Tarasoff rule.[22,23] Varying across states, standards include duties to protect or warn or permission to warn individuals, groups of people, or even structures. Some jurisdictions have specifically stated that clinicians have no such duties. A periodically updated list of the specific legal standards by state, including links to pertinent case law or statute, is accessible at http://www.ncsl.org/research/health/mental-health-professionals-duty-to-warn.aspx.

Professional organizations have also proffered guidance on responding to threats to third parties. The American Medical Association (AMA) identifies a duty to protect with parameters quite similar to the Tarasoff rule in Ethics Opinion 5.05:

When a patient threatens to inflict serious physical harm to another person or to him or herself and there is a reasonable probability that the patient may carry out the threat, the physician should take reasonable precautions for the protection of the intended victim, which may include notification of law enforcement authorities.[24]

The 2013 American Psychiatric Association (APA) Principles of Medical Ethics with Annotations for Psychiatry permits breach of confidentiality in situations in which "the risk of danger is deemed to be significant."[25] Thus, the APA identifies a permission to warn. Psychiatrists are arguably expected to comply with AMA as well as APA ethics standards, thus creating the dual obligation of a duty to protect and permission to warn.

Professional ethics standards are particularly relevant to this issue due to the Health Insurance Portability and Accountability Act (HIPAA) Privacy Rule that permits warning when it is in accordance with either appropriate local legal standards or professional ethical standards.[26,27] Most mental health professional organizations offer some type of guidance on this issue within their ethical standards.

DUTIES TO THIRD PARTIES: FITTING THE LEGAL AND ETHICAL PARAMETERS TO CLINICAL CARE

Ultimately, emergency mental health professionals may find strict analysis by applicable legal standards to be unsatisfying. At times this is due to the vagueness of the available legal standard or a mismatch between the specific facts of the clinical case and the rule or facts of the precedential statute or court ruling. Careful and well-documented clinical judgment in such circumstances is advised. Clinicians should consider that such dilemmas inevitably involve 2 paths with risks that can differ substantially in ways that may not be easily quantifiable; often the perception that 1 path is risk-free is actually misperception with risks unrecognized or intentionally ignored and minimized. Timely consultation with other psychiatrists, administration, legal counsel, or ethicists may be useful.

Assuming a worst-case scenario for either alternative, the choice may actually be somewhat simple. That is, if we assume warning or involuntary admission will lead to a lawsuit by the patient and failure to do so leads to an attack and subsequent lawsuit by the victim or victim's survivors, the choice may be somewhat easier. Here, the choice is between defending a case due to transient violation of the patient's rights versus defending a case due to potentially deadly harm. All things being equal, many would rather defend, or even pay the cost of settlement, for the former rather than the latter.

Clinicians should always be mindful that warning does not necessarily equate to protection and a target may still be at risk, or even be placed at greater risk, after a warning. Warnings should be delivered with attention paid to the emotional impact on the target, and linkage to victim advocacy, law enforcement, and other appropriate supports should be considered. Although warnings are usually delivered to an identified target, some jurisdictions provide for warnings to law enforcement as well.

FIREARMS AND PSYCHIATRIC EMERGENCIES

Contrary to public perception, violence and homicide in America have decreased in the past 20 to 25 years. Homicide has decreased approximately 50%, firearm crimes are down by approximately 75%. However, the United States continues to see firearm use in 20,000 firearm suicides, 10,000 to 12,000 homicides, 60,000 to 70,000 nonlethal shootings, and more than 450,000 other violent incidents yearly.[28,29] The United States has a firearm homicide rate 25 times higher and a firearm suicide rate 8 times higher compared with other developed nations.[30] It should be noted that media-driven perceptions of frequent mass shootings or an outsized role of mental illness in violence is false.[31,32] That said, and political rhetoric notwithstanding, there is no serious scientific debate about the appropriateness of physicians exploring and counseling about firearm access and safety.[33–38]

Unfortunately there is limited evidence-based, well-publicized guidance in effectively evaluating firearm access and safety counseling by physicians.[39] Not surprisingly then, many psychiatrists and emergency physicians report infrequently asking about access or counseling on secure storage even when working with suicidal patients.[40,41] Counseling patients and family members about firearms is complex. Firearm ownership and access may be a priority consideration for the clinician, but for the patient it may be seen as a civil right and one under threat. Engaging a patient or family member on this topic is challenging and often fraught with additional challenges due to cultural divide issues. Early efforts to develop a motivational interviewing, culturally sensitive approach to this challenge is under way.[42,43] Effective assessment and safety counseling for firearms is an emerging and vital clinical competency.[41]

SUMMARY

Violence in the ED is a significant problem, impacting health care workers in this setting and causing significant difficulties in management. The nature of the ED setting often portends an increased risk of violence. Further, patients may present with violent ideation or threats, often necessitating additional duties. A risk assessment can be used as part of clinical judgment in these situations to assist with disposition and management. Additional approaches in the ED and at broader levels can be taken to reduce the risk for patients, third-party targets of violent ideation, and staff in the ED.

REFERENCES

1. Occupational Health and Safety Administration. (n.d.). Workplace violence in healthcare. United States department of labor. Available at: https://www.osha.gov/Publications/OSHA3826.pdf. Accessed April 30, 2016.
2. American College of Emergency Physicians. (n.d.). American College of Emergency Physicians - fact sheets. Available at: http://newsroom.acep.org/fact_sheets?item=30010. Accessed April 30, 2016.

3. Emergency Nurses Association. Emergency department violence surveillance study. 2011. Available at: https://www.ena.org/practice-research/research/Documents/ENAEDVSReportNovember2011.pdf. Accessed April 30, 2016.

4. Gates DM, Ross CS, McQueen L. Violence against emergency department workers. J Emerg Med 2006;31(3):331–7.

5. Turkcuer I. Assessment of the relation of violence and burnout among physicians working in the emergency departments in Turkey. Ulus Travma Acil Cerrahi Derg 2015;21(3):175–81.

6. Kowalenko T, Gates D, Gillespie GL, et al. Prospective study of violence against ED workers. Am J Emerg Med 2013;31(1):197–205.

7. Gillespie GL, Gates DM, Berry P. Stressful incidents of physical violence against emergency nurses. Online J Issues Nurs 2013;18(1):2.

8. Norko MA, Baranoski MV. The prediction of violence; detection of dangerousness. Brief Treat Crisis Interv 2008;8(1):73–91.

9. Davison S. The management of violence in general psychiatry. Adv Psychiatr Treat 2005;11:362–70.

10. Singh JP, Grann M, Fazel S. A comparative study of violence risk assessment tools: a systematic review and metaregression analysis of 68 studies involving 25,980 participants. Clin Psychol Rev 2011;31(3):499–513.

11. Buchanan A, Binder R, Norko M, et al. Psychiatric violence risk assessment. Am J Psychiatry 2012;169(3):340.

12. Kowalenko T, Cunningham R, Sachs CJ, et al. Workplace violence in emergency medicine: current knowledge and future directions. J Emerg Med 2012;43(3):523–31.

13. Byatt N, Glick R. Safety in the psychiatric emergency service. In: Glick RL, Berlin JS, Fishkind AB, et al, editors. Emergency psychiatry: principles and practice. Philadelphia: Lippincott Williams & Wilkins; 2008. p. 33–44.

14. Holloman GH, Zeller SL. Overview of project beta: best practices in evaluation and treatment of agitation. West J Emerg Med 2012;13(1):1–2.

15. Knox DK, Holloman GH. Use and avoidance of seclusion and restraint: consensus statement of the American Association for Emergency Psychiatry Project Beta seclusion and restraint workgroup. West J Emerg Med 2012;13(1):35–40.

16. Nordstrom K, Zun LS, Wilson MP, et al. Medical evaluation and triage of the agitated patient: consensus statement of the American Association for Emergency Psychiatry Project Beta medical evaluation workgroup. West J Emerg Med 2012;13(1):3–10.

17. Richmond JS, Berlin JS, Fishkind AB, et al. Verbal de-escalation of the agitated patient: consensus statement of the American Association for Emergency Psychiatry Project Beta de-escalation workgroup. West J Emerg Med 2012;13(1):17–25.

18. Stowell KR, Florence P, Harman HJ, et al. Psychiatric evaluation of the agitated patient: consensus statement of the American Association for Emergency Psychiatry Project Beta psychiatric evaluation workgroup. West J Emerg Med 2012;13(1):11–6.

19. Wilson MP, Pepper D, Currier GW, et al. The psychopharmacology of agitation: consensus statement of the American Association for Emergency Psychiatry Project Beta psychopharmacology workgroup. West J Emerg Med 2012;13(1):26–34.

20. McNamara R, Yu DK, Kelly JJ. Public perception of safety and metal detectors in an urban emergency department. West J Emerg Med 1997;15(1):40–2.

21. Tarasoff v. Regents of the University of California, 551 P.2d 334 (Cal. 1976).

22. Werth J, Welfel E, Benjamin G. The duty to protect: ethical, legal, and professional considerations for mental health professionals. Washington, DC: American Psychological Association; 2009.

23. National Conference of State Legislatures. Mental Health Professionals' Duty to Warn, September 28, 2015. Available at: http://www.ncsl.org/research/health/mentalhealth-professionals-duty-to-warn.aspx. Accessed April 30, 2016.

24. American Medical Association. (n.d.). Opinion 5.05-Confidentiality. Available at: http://www.ama-assn.org/ama/pub/physician-resources/medical-ethics/code-medical-ethics/opinion505.page. Accessed April 30, 2016.

25. American Psychiatric Association. The principles of medical ethics with annotations especially applicable to psychiatry. 2013.

26. Code of Federal Regulations. Title 45: public welfare. College Park, MD: National Archives and Records Administration; 2004.

27. Rodriguez L. Message to our nation's healthcare providers from the US Department of Health and Human Services. 2013. Available at: http://www.hhs.gov/about/news/2013/01/16/statement-from-hhs-secretary-sebelius-on-presidents-sandy-hook-response-plan.html. Accessed April 30, 2016.

28. Fowler KA, Dahlberg LL, Haileyesus T, et al. Firearm injuries in the United States. Prev Med 2015;79:5–14.

29. Truman J, Langton L. Criminal victimization, 2014. Washington, DC: US Department of Justice; 2015. Available at: http://www.bjs.gov/content/pub/pdf/cv14.pdf. Accessed April 30, 2016.

30. Grinshteyn E, Hemenway D. Violent death rates: the US compared with other high-income OECD countries, 2010. Am J Med 2016;129(3):266–73.

31. Fisher CE, Lieberman JA. Getting the facts straight about gun violence and mental illness: putting compassion before fear. Ann Intern Med 2013;159(6):423–4.

32. Metzl JM, MacLeish KT. Mental illness, mass shootings, and the politics of American firearms. Am J Public Health 2015;105(2):240–9.

33. Appelbaum PS. Public safety, mental disorders, and guns. JAMA Psychiatry 2013;70(6):565–6.

34. Bonnie RJ, Appelbaum PS, Pinals DA. The evolving position of the American Psychiatric Association on Firearm Policy (1993-2014): evolving APA position on firearm policy. Behav Sci Law 2015;33(2–3):178–85.

35. Brent DA, Miller MJ, Loeber R, et al. Ending the silence on gun violence. J Am Acad Child Adolesc Psychiatry 2013;52(4):333–8.

36. Gold LH. Gun violence: psychiatry, risk assessment, and social policy. J Am Acad Psychiatry Law 2013;41(3):337–43.

37. Laine C, Taichman DB, Mulrow C, et al. A resolution for physicians: time to focus on the public health threat of gun violence. Ann Intern Med 2013; 158(6):493–4.

38. Pinals DA, Appelbaum PS, Bonnie RJ, et al. Resource document on access to firearms by people with mental disorders: resource document on access to firearms by people with mental disorders. Behav Sci Law 2015;33(2–3):186–94.

39. Roszko PJD, Ameli J, Carter PM, et al. Clinician attitudes, screening practices, and interventions to reduce firearm-related injury. Epidemiol Rev 2016;38(1):87–110.

40. Betz ME, Wintemute GJ. Physician counseling on firearm safety: a new kind of cultural competence. JAMA 2015;314(5):449–50.

41. Price JH, Kinnison A, Dake JA, et al. Psychiatrists' practices and perceptions regarding anticipatory guidance on firearms. Am J Prev Med 2007;33(5):370–3.

42. Ghandi T. Do you have access to guns? Am J Psychiatry Resid J 2016;11(1): 3–4.
43. Rozel J, Soliman L, Jain A. The gun talk: how to talk to patients and families about guns and gun safety. Presented at the Institute on Psychiatric Services. New York, October 9–11, 2015.

Inpatient Violence

Kayla Fisher, MD, JD[a,b],*

KEYWORDS

- Inpatient violence • Risk factors • Inpatient aggression

KEY POINTS

- Research indicates that 25% to 35% of psychiatric inpatients engage in violence.
- Past violence best predicts future violence.
- Long-term risks of violence include a history of violence, psychotic disorders, substance use disorder, personality disorders, intellectual disabilities, violent suicide attempts, and neurologic abnormalities.
- Short-term risks include recent violence or threats of violence, positive symptoms of a psychotic disorder, irritability, hostility, psychomotor agitation, and a poor therapeutic alliance.
- A small percentage of patients account for approximately half of the violence and more than half of all serious injuries.
- Determining whether violence flows from psychosis, impulsivity, or predatory characteristics helps guide interventions.
- A highly structured unit with strong psychiatric leadership, free of excessive noise and crowding, with adequate nursing staff helps decrease violence.

INTRODUCTION

Inpatient violence constitutes a major concern for psychiatric hospitals and institutions. Research indicates that 25% to 35% of inpatients exhibit violent behavior during their hospitalization.[1,2] The consequences of this violence affect both staff and patients and include psychological suffering and physical injury.[3,4] Victimized staff often experience decreased productivity, diminished work satisfaction,[4] and emotional distress,[5] whereas patients experience significant disruption of the treatment environment and a negative atmosphere in the milieu.[2]

Inpatient violence can also lead to feelings of anger and helplessness on the psychiatric unit.[6] As a result, staff frequently manage violent behavior by using seclusion and restraint, which, in themselves, pose physical and psychological risks.[7,8] Although

Disclosures: None.
[a] Patton State Hospital, California Department of State Hospitals, 3102 East Highland Avenue, Patton, CA 92369, USA; [b] Department of Psychiatry, University of California, Riverside School of Medicine, Riverside, CA 92521, USA
* Patton State Hospital, California Department of State Hospitals, 3102 East Highland Avenue, Patton, CA 92369.
E-mail address: Kayla.Fisher@dsh.ca.gov

violence and aggressive behavior have presented significant challenges for psychiatric facilities for decades,[9] violence should not be thought of as inevitable.[10] By determining the causes of violence and embarking on solutions, we can focus on reducing inpatient violence and, work towards, eliminating it altogether.

VICTIMS OF INPATIENT VIOLENCE

Patients and staff entering a psychiatric unit often express concerns about whether they will become victims of violence. Although aggressive patients target both staff and peers, existing research provides conflicting data as to which group receives more assaults. Of staff members who are victimized, nursing staff is the group most frequently targeted by violent patients.[11] Although research remains inconclusive as to whether patients most often victimize female or male staff across all inpatient settings, studies conducted in select state hospitals found that female staff is more likely to be assaulted.[12,13] A 2003 study found that aggressive incidents tended to involve victims and perpetrators of the same sex. In contrast, violent patients exhibiting sexual aggression only targeted female staff.[2] In a 2006 study, Daffern and colleagues[14] found, despite staff perceptions to the contrary, no correlation existed between the proportions of men on duty and frequency of violence. A strong correlation does exist, however, among age, experience, training, and inpatient violence. Although being of younger age constitutes an increased risk, staff possessing experience and additional formal training have less risk of victimization.[15]

ENVIRONMENTAL FACTORS ASSOCIATED WITH INCREASED INPATIENT VIOLENCE

To lessen the likelihood of violence in the inpatient setting, the treating environment must be carefully designed and monitored. Studies find an association between environmental conditions and psychiatric inpatient violence.

The following are associated with an increase in psychiatric inpatient violence:

- High acuity units[2]
- Shift change[16,17]
- Meal time[16,17]
- Medication time[18]
- Narrow hallways[19]
- Crowded areas[19]
- More psychotic patients on units[20]
- Excessive noise[13,15,21]
- Few nursing staff[22]
- Substitute nursing staff[23]
- Absence of strong psychiatric leadership[24]
- Poorly defined staff roles[24]
- Lack of unit structure[24]
- Absence of predictable routines[24]
- Lack of therapeutic alliance between staff and patients[24]
- Caffeinated beverages[25]

IDENTIFYING VIOLENT PATIENTS

Past violence best predicts future violence just as past behavior is the best predictor of future behavior.[26] The best way to evaluate past behavior is by a careful review of a patient's history. A violent patient often has a history of violence reflected in their hospital chart or criminal record.[14,21,27,28] As expected, involuntarily admitted patients also possess a higher risk of violence than voluntarily admitted ones, as recent violence or the threat of violence often constitutes the substantiation for an involuntary admission.[29] Of the involuntarily admitted patients, those deemed "dangerous to others" show more violent behavior within the first 72 hours of their hospitalization compared with patients committed to the hospital for other reasons.[30] Patients with a history of past violent suicide attempts also carry an increased risk of violence.[31,32] Therefore, a careful review of historical factors, including criminal charges, hospital charts, and jail records, provides important information with regard to a patient's likelihood of violence and insight into safeguards needed.

Of the violent patients, a subset exists of extreme offenders. This small group of especially violent patients accounts for most of the inpatient violence and the most serious injuries.[33] In one study, for example, only 5% of the patients accounted for approximately half of the violent behavior and more than half of the serious injuries.[34] These patients inflict serious injuries at a rate 10 times greater than that of other violent patients. These recidivist violent patients can be of either gender. Convit and colleagues[34] found that women who displayed this repeatedly violent behavior were more likely to present with organic brain disorder or personality disorder than nonrecidivist women. Recidivist men, however, more often carried the diagnosis of schizophrenia than did nonrecidivist men.[34]

Although gender rates of violence differ in the community, research indicates otherwise for the inpatient setting. In psychiatric institutions, women equal men in their risk of exhibiting violent behavior,[35] even though men engage in more violence in the community.[36] Studies suggest that younger patients exhibit more violence than older patients.[23] Similarly, research in prisons found increased violence in younger populations, whereas a housing unit with a heterogeneous mix of ages experienced decreased aggression rates.[37,38]

The patient's developmental factors can also impact their likelihood of inpatient aggression. A history of truancy, foster care, or childhood physical abuse increases the likelihood of aggression. Additionally, a history of parental substance use disorder or psychiatric illness increases the risk that the patient will act violently.[31,39]

Violence can flow from substance intoxication, substance withdrawal, or physical conditions.[40,41] In addition to the short-term risk of violence posed by substance intoxication or withdrawal, patients with a history of substance-use disorders present with an increased long-term risk for inpatient violence.[27,42–44] Frontal lobe deficits, dementia, psychomotor agitation, akathisia, and physical discomfort or pain all increase a patient's risk of behaving violently. Delirium, sleep issues, complex partial seizures, and thyroid disease can also lead to increased aggression.[40,41] Additionally, head injuries and temporal lobe lesions can increase a patient's acts of violence.[45]

PSYCHIATRIC SYMPTOMS OF VIOLENT PATIENTS

Aggressive patients constitute a heterogeneous group. Research indicates the importance of categorizing violence according to the underlying psychiatric motive to target interventions. Three primary psychiatric etiologies account for the violence on inpatient settings—problems with impulse control, symptoms of psychosis, and predatory characteristics.[26,46]

Impulsivity

Most of the violence on inpatient settings flows from impulsivity. The impulsivity associated with violence is accompanied by emotional hypersensitivity, exaggerated threat perception, hyperreactivity to stimuli, or autonomic arousal.[41] The characteristics of this impulsive aggression involve a reactive or emotional response with a loss of behavioral control coupled with a failure to consider consequences.[41]

Patients who act aggressively secondary to impulsivity most often target staff.[47] Assaults secondary to impulsivity often arise from staff attempts to change a patient's unwanted behavior. Other times, these assaults occur when staff refuse a patient's request.[47]

Impulsivity can arise from various psychiatric diagnoses. Substance use disorders have a strong association with impulsivity. Other diagnoses linked with impulsivity include schizophrenia spectrum disorders, cognitive disorders, attention deficit hyperactivity disorder, intermittent explosive disorder, traumatic brain injury, bipolar disorder, depressive disorders, posttraumatic spectrum disorder, antisocial personality disorder, and borderline personality disorder.[41]

Psychosis

As might be expected, the presence of psychosis increases a patient's likelihood of acting violently. Psychotic assaults make up approximately 17% of the inpatient aggression, with other patients most often being the victims.[47] Diagnoses associated with psychotic aggression include the schizophrenia spectrum disorders and bipolar spectrum disorders. Other diagnoses that can result in psychotic aggression include major cognitive disorders such as Alzheimer's disease, vascular dementia, traumatic brain injury, and major cognitive disorder with Lewy bodies.[41]

Of the psychotic patients, patients with paranoid delusions or command hallucinations suffer from a particularly high risk of engaging in violent behavior. In fact, patients that experience command hallucinations are twice as likely to assault when compared with patients who do not have this symptom.[48] Factors that increase the likelihood that the patient will act on the command hallucination include hearing a familiar voice in the hallucination, experiencing an associated delusion, and the absence of coping strategies.[49] Thought disorders, which can cause a patient to misinterpret the stimuli in their environment, also elevate risk of aggressive activity.[41,50]

Predatory Violence

Predatory violence typically occurs without any warning and is difficult to predict or prevent.[51] Patients with predatory characteristics execute planned, organized, goal-directed, assaults while remaining emotionally detached. These acts account for approximately 29% of the inpatient violence. Predatory patients most commonly target other patients.[50] These aggressors engage in purposeful, planned behavior to attain one of their personal goals.[41] The clinical findings of psychopathy or an antisocial personality disorder serve as long-term risk factors for this predatory aggression.[51]

SHORT-TERM VERSUS LONG-TERM RISK FACTORS FOR VIOLENCE

Risk factors for violence are commonly grouped into short-term risk factors, which help predict violence in the upcoming few days, and long-term risk factors. Awareness of which risk factors constitute short-term versus long-term risk provides critical information to guide treatment interventions. Clinical risk factors, rather than demographic risk factors, best predict violence in the short-term timeframe.[52] These short-term risks for inpatient aggression include:

- Recent physical violence or a threat of violence (most predictive)[53,54]
- Severe positive symptoms/thought disorder[39,55,56]

- Irritability or hostility[57]
- Psychomotor agitation[58,59]
- Lack of a therapeutic alliance with staff[26,60]

As previously discussed, past violence is the best long-term predictor of inpatient violence.[61] Other long-term risk factors include violent suicide attempts,[31,33] psychotic disorders, substance use disorder, intellectual disabilities,[39,62–65] antisocial and borderline personality disorders,[33,64–66] a history of truancy, childhood physical abuse, foster placement,[31,39] and neurologic abnormalities.[26,67–69]

GENERAL STRATEGIES TO MINIMIZE PSYCHIATRIC INPATIENT VIOLENCE

Using the research available, much can be done to provide for safer inpatient psychiatric settings. These strategies include:

- Supply units with adequate numbers of nursing staff.
- Minimize reliance on temporary or substitute nursing staff.
- Avoid overcrowded units and areas.
- Consider extra monitoring during unit transition times.
- Avoid excessive noise on psychiatric unit.
- Train staff on skills to develop strong therapeutic alliances with patients.
- Provide structure with therapeutic activities and clearly defined staff roles.
- Educate staff to identify early signs of agitation and use de-escalation techniques.
- Maintain strong psychiatric leadership on the unit.
- Prescribe and administer medications as clinically indicated to target underlying etiology of violence.
- Gear psychosocial treatments to target underlying etiology of violence—impulsivity, psychosis, or predatory characteristics.
- Employ one-to-one staff observation as clinically indicated.
- Use seclusion and restraint when clinically indicated as the least restrictive means to provide safety.
- After a violent incident, use debriefing sessions to glean vital information for use in developing additional approaches to prevent subsequent violence.

STRATEGIES FOR TYPE-SPECIFIC VIOLENCE

In addition to the general strategies to decrease inpatient violence listed above, certain strategies can be used to target the specific cause of the aggressive behavior. Once these strategies are identified, it is often helpful for clinicians to write a formal violence reduction plan, taking into account the specific etiologies driving the violence risk.[70]

Strategies to Minimize Violence Driven by Impulsivity

When impulsivity drives the violence, careful observation of the patient for escalating behaviors aids clinicians in using de-escalation techniques at the first opportunity. Additionally, because most of the violence from impulsive patients arises after an aversive stimulus, clinicians need to use skill in their interactions with these patients to prevent them from escalating.[26,71] Pre-assaultive behaviors often include verbal abuse, a raised voice, swearing, and standing uncomfortably close.[59]

Before using de-escalation techniques, first make sure sufficient personal space exists between you and the patient, while locating an escape route. Summon help, if needed. To de-escalate the patient, talk with the patient, using a calm voice and find out what the patient is upset about. Try to understand the patient's perspective and agree with them, if possible. Offer the patient choices as to next behaviors they might engage in—taking medication, listening to music, or talking more to staff. Be respectful of the patient and avoid arguing with them. If possible, accompany the patient to a calmer space where they can relax.[26]

Strategies to Minimize Violence from Psychosis

When violence flows from psychosis, patients require monitoring for increased paranoid or persecutory delusions.[26] When paranoid fear keeps building in a crescendolike manner, such patients pose a threat even though they may not voice a threat.[70] It is also important to especially monitor patients at the onset of their psychotic episode, as the median length of time between the onset of such an episode and violence is 30 days.[72]

Various published psychopharmacologic approaches advise physicians on how to target psychiatric symptoms that give rise to violence. The California State Hospital Violence Assessment and Treatment Guidelines[26] is one set of "comprehensive guidelines for the assessment and treatment of violence and aggression of various etiologies" that "employ off-label prescribing practices."[26] Although useful, the guidelines emphasize that they do not remove a physician's responsibility to make individual medication and other treatment decisions, taking into account the patient's particular risks and benefits.

Strategies to Minimize Violence from Predatory Aggression

In situations in which aggression results from predatory characteristics flowing from antisocial personality disorder or psychopathology, efforts that result in the patient assuming responsibility for their behavior serve an important therapeutic function.[26] Some institutions have implemented models that allow for the prosecution of patients for presumptively criminally acts.[73] Although still controversial, many argue that criminal prosecution sets firm limits on antisocial behavior and results in positive change.[74,75] Justifications for prosecution of assaultive patients include (1) retribution, (2) deterrence, (3) incapacitation through incarceration, and (4) rehabilitation.[74] Just as clinicians possess a "Tarasoff" duty to protect third parties, the US Supreme Court found constitutional justification for imposing like duties on inpatient clinicians to provide safe conditions for patients.[73,76,77] Some have argued that when patients engage in planned aggression to meet their own needs and such acts go unpunished, the aggressive behavior may be positively reinforced. If psychiatric institutions allow such behavior, the patient may end up believing there will not be serious consequences for their acts of violence. Such patients can then have more difficulty when they go back into society.[26,78]

When a facility has an ability to pursue prosecution of violence, serving notice of this at the time of admission may deter such violence from occurring. This can be done when providing the patient with their rights and responsibilities by adding a statement that failure to follow the rules of the hospital and to show respect for the law could result in criminal charges.[26] Violence can also be mitigated by informing an already assaultive patient that the hospital intends to pursue prosecution, as this may decrease future violence from the patient.[79]

ARCHITECTURAL STRATEGIES TO REDUCE VIOLENCE

In general, psychiatric hospital designs that minimize stress reduce aggression.[80,81] Designs that minimize crowding, provide access to nature or other stress reducing features, foster a degree of privacy, minimize noise, and allow for a sense of control all reduce aggression.[80,81] Research on prisons and residential settings indicates that there is a correlation between the number of persons sharing a bedroom, bathroom, or cell and the number of disagreements with roommates, illness complaints, and social withdrawal.[82–84] In keeping with these findings, some recent high-security psychiatric hospitals have been designed with single "en suite" rooms.[85] Other design features that may reduce violence include multiple multipurpose rooms that allow for smaller group sizes, spacious day rooms with movable seating that allows patients to maintain personal space, sound-absorbing surfaces to reduce noise, windows that allow nature views, a garden accessible to patients, art with nature scenes, and exposure to natural light.[86]

In designing the nursing unit, architects are met with the challenge of providing for staff safety while allowing for adequate auditory and visual monitoring and promoting a therapeutic environment in which patients are treated with dignity. Some successful designs include using a combination of partition height and counter depth to prevent patient access to the nursing side. Clear partitions specially designed to resist breakage can also be used to help maintain this balance between the needs of maintaining therapeutic milieu, clinical monitoring, and safety.[87]

SECURITY PERSONNEL, WEAPONS, AND VIOLENCE

According to a 2014 national survey,[88] the use of hospital security personnel carrying handguns and Tasers has doubled in the last 3 years. Currently, 52% of hospitals have security personnel carrying handguns and 47% of hospitals have security personnel using Tasers. Only 12% of hospitals use K-9 units and 52% use pepper spray. Although an increase of violence risk was noted with those hospitals that use pepper spray, hospitals that use K-9 units show a decreased risk for violence. Those hospitals that allow security personnel to carry handguns show a decreased risk of physical assaults but a slight increased risk of overall violent events. Interestingly, this study found that hospitals allowing the use of Tasers had a 41% lower risk of physical assault, even when controlling for other measures such as hospital characteristics and availability of other weapons.[88]

Although clinicians working on psychiatric units may favor increased presence of security personnel, they are often opposed to the presence of weapons.[89] Over the last several years, more than a dozen incidents were reported of patients who were killed or injured by hospital security personnel.[89,90] Although many of these security personnel have military or law enforcement backgrounds, security experts emphasize that it takes a different mindset to work in a health care setting.[89] In fact, state psychiatric hospitals do not typically allow Tasers or guns on their premises. For facilities that decide to use Tasers or other weapons, proper training of security personnel is essential.[88]

SUMMARY

Although violence remains a significant challenge for psychiatric inpatient settings, many interventions exist that decrease the likelihood of violence. By taking time to investigate a patient's history and possible motivations for violence, treatment and environmental strategies can be used to target the potential for violence before it occurs. This information, coupled with the clinical findings and targeted treatments, can be useful in preventing inpatient violence.

REFERENCES

1. Arango C, Calcedo Barba A, Gonzalez-Salvador T, et al. Violence in inpatients with schizophrenia: a prospective study. Schizophr Bull 1999;25:493–503.
2. Daffern M, Mayer MM, Martin T. A preliminary investigation into patterns of aggression in an Australian forensic psychiatric hospital. J Forensic Psychiatry Psychol 2003;14:67–84.
3. Flannery R. Repetitively assaultive psychiatric patients: review of published findings, 1978-2001. Psychiatr Q 2002;73:229–37.
4. Johnson ME. Violence on inpatient psychiatric units: state of the science. J Am Psychiatr Nurses Assoc 2004;10:113–21.
5. Quintal SA. Violence against psychiatric nurses, an untreated epidemic? J Psychosoc Nurs Ment Health Serv 2002;40:46–53.
6. Menckel E, Viitaxara E. Threats and violence in Swedish care and welfare— Magnitude of the problem and impact on municipal personnel. Scand J Caring Sci 2002;16(4):376–85.
7. Frueh B, Knapp R, Cusack K, et al. Patients' reports of traumatic or harmful experiences within the psychiatric setting. Psychiatr Serv 2005;56:1123–33.
8. Kaltiala-Heino R, Tuohimaki C, Korkeila J, et al. Reasons for using seclusion and restraint in psychiatric inpatient care. Int J Law Psychiatry 2003;26:139–49.
9. Needham I, Abderhaldern C, Meer R, et al. The effectiveness of two interventions in the management of patient violence in acute mental inpatient settings: report on a pilot study. J Psychiatr Ment Health Nurs 2004;11:595–601.
10. Welsh E, Bader S, Evans S. Situational variables related to aggression in institutional settings. Aggress Violent Behav 2013;18:792–6.
11. Tardiff K. The risk of being attacked by patients: who, how often, and where?. In: Eichelman B, Hartwig A, editors. Patient violence and the clinician. Washington, DC: American Psychiatric Press; 1995. p. 13–32.
12. Flannery R, Farley E, Rego S, et al. Characteristics of staff victims of psychiatric patient assaults: 15-year analysis of the Assaulted Staff Action Program (ASAP). Psychiatry Q 2007;78:25–37.
13. Flannery R, Hanson MD, Penk W. Risk factors for psychiatric inpatient assaults on staff. J Ment Health Adm 1994;21:24–31.
14. Daffern M, Mayer M, Martin T. Staff gender ration and aggression in a forensic psychiatric hospital. Int J Ment Health Nurs 2006;15:93–9.
15. Flannery R, Staffieri A, Hildum S, et al. The violence triad and common single precipitants to psychiatric patient assaults on staff: 16-year analysis of the assaulted staff program. Psychiatry Q 2011;82:85–93.
16. Balderston C, Negley E, Kelly G, et al. Data-based interventions to reduce assaults by geriatric inpatients. Hosp Community Psychiatry 1990;41:447–9.
17. Weizmann-Henelius G, Suutala H. Violence in a Finnish forensic psychiatric hospital. Nord J Psychiatry 2000;54:269–73.
18. Bader S, Evans S, Welsh E. Aggression Among Psychiatric Inpatients: The Relationship Between Time, Place, Victims, and Severity Ratings. J Am Psychiatr Nurses Assoc 2014;20(3):179–86.
19. Chou K, Lu R, Mao W. Factors relevant to patient assaultive behavior and assault in acute inpatient psychiatric units in Taiwan. Arch Psychiatr Nurs 2002;16:187–95.
20. Palmstierna T, Huitfeldt B, Wistedt B. The relationship of crowding and aggressive behavior on a psychiatric intensive care unit. Hosp Community Psychiatry 1991;42:1237–40.

21. Flannery R, Peterson B, Walker A. Precipitants of elderly psychiatric patient assaults on staff: preliminary empirical inquiry. Psychiatr Q 2005;76:167–75.
22. Lanza M, Kayne H, Hicks C, et al. Environmental characteristics related to patient assault. Issues Ment Health Nurs 1994;15:319–35.
23. James D, Fineber N, Shah A, et al. An increase in violence on an acute psychiatric ward: a study of associated factors. Br J Psychiatry 1990;156:846–52.
24. Katz P, Kirkland F. Violence and social structure on mental hospital wards. Psychiatry 1990;53:262–77.
25. Zaslove M, Beal M, McKinney R. Changes in behaviors of inpatients after a ban on the sale of caffeinated drinks. Hosp Community Psychiatry 1991;42(1):84–5.
26. Quanbeck C, McDermott B. Inpatient Settings. In: Simon R, Tardiff K, editors. Textbook of violence assessment and Management. Washington, DC: American Psychiatric Association Publishing, Inc; 2008. p. 259–70.
27. El-Badri S, Mellsop G. Aggressive behaviour in an acute general adult psychiatric unit. Psychiatr Bull 2006;30:166–8.
28. Grassi L, Peron L, Marangoni C, et al. Characteristics of violent behavior in acute psychiatric in-patients: a 5-year Italian study. Acta Psychiatr Scand 2001;104: 273–9.
29. Nijman H, Allertz W, Merckelbach H, et al. Aggressive behavior on an acute psychiatric admissions ward. Eur J Psychiatry 1997;11:106–14.
30. McNiel D, Binder R. Predictive validity judgments of dangerousness in emergency civil commitment. Am J Psychiatry 1987;144:197–200.
31. Convit A, Jaegar J, Lin S, et al. Predicting assaultiveness in psychiatric inpatients: a pilot study. Hosp Community Psychiatry 1988;39:429–34.
32. Soliman A, Reza H. Risk factors and correlates of violence among acutely ill adult psychiatric inpatients. Psychiatr Serv 2001;52:75–80.
33. Kraus J, Sheitman B. Characteristics of violent behavior in a large state psychiatric hospital. Psychiatr Serv 2004;55:183–5.
34. Convit A, Isay D, Otis D, et al. Characteristics of repeatedly assaultive psychiatric inpatients. Hosp Community Psychiatry 1990;41:1112–5.
35. Lam J, McNiel D, Binder R. The relationship between patients' gender and violence leading to staff injuries. Psychiatr Serv 2000;51:1167–70.
36. Swanson J, Holzer C, Ganju V, et al. Violence and psychiatric disorder in the community: evidence from the Epidemiologic Catchment Area surveys. Hosp Community Psychiatry 1990;41:761–70.
37. Ekland-Olson S, Barrick D, Cohen L. Prison overcrowding and disciplinary problems: an analysis of the Texas prison system. J Appl Behav Sci 1983;19(2): 163–92.
38. Mabli J, Holley C, Patrick J, et al. Age and prison violence: increasing age heterogeneity as a violence-reducing strategy in prisons. Crim Justice Behav 1979;6(2): 175–86.
39. Hoptman M, Yates K, Patalinjug M, et al. Clinical prediction of assaultive behavior among male psychiatric patients at a maximum-security forensic facility. Psychiatr Serv 1999;50:1461–6.
40. Hankin C, Bronstone A, Koran L. Agitation in the inpatient psychiatric setting: a review of clinical presentation, burden, and treatment. J Psychiatr Pract 2011; 17(3):170–85.
41. Stahl S, Morrissette D, Cummings M, et al. California State Hospital Violence Assessment and Treatment (Cal-VAT) guidelines. CNS Spectr 2014;19(5):449–65.
42. Barlow I, Grenyet B, Ilkiw-Lavalle O. Prevalence and precipitants of aggression in psychiatric inpatient units. Aust N Z J Psychiatry 2000;34:967–74.

43. Daffern M, Howells K, Ogloff J. The interaction between individual characteristics and the function of aggression in forensic psychiatric inpatients. Psychiatry Psychol L 2007;14:17–25.
44. Myers K, Dunner D. Self and other directed violence on a closed acute-care ward. Psychiatr Q 1984;56:178–88.
45. Volavka J. Neurobiology of violence. Washington, DC: American Psychiatric Publishing, Inc; 2002.
46. Nolan K, Czobor P, Roy B, et al. Characteristics of assaultive behavior among psychiatric inpatients. Psychiatr Serv 2003;54:1012–6.
47. Quanbeck C, McDermott B, Lam J, et al. Categorization of aggressive acts committed by chronically assaultive state hospital patients. Psychiatr Serv 2007;58:521–8.
48. McNiel D, Eisner J, Binder R. The relationship between command hallucinations and violence. Psychiatr Serv 2000;51:1288–92.
49. Cheung P, Schweitzer I, Crowley K, et al. Violence in schizophrenia: role of hallucinations and delusions. Schizophr Res 1997;26:181–90.
50. Volavka J, Citrome L. Pathways to aggression in schizophrenia affect results of treatment. Schizophr Bull 2011;37(5):921–9.
51. Meloy J. The prediction of violence in outpatient psychotherapy. Am J Psychotherapy 1987;41:38–45.
52. McNiel D, Gregory A, Lam J, et al. Utility of decision support tools for assessing acute risk of violence. J Consult Clin Psychol 2003;71:945–53.
53. McNiel D, Binder R. Relationship between preadmission threats and later violent behavior by acute psychiatric inpatients. Hosp Community Psychiatry 1989;40:605–8.
54. McNiel D, Binder R, Greenfield T. Predictors of violence in civilly committed acute psychiatric patients. Am J Psychiatry 1988;145:965–70.
55. Krakowski M, Czobor P, Chou J. Course of violence in patients with schizophrenia: relationship to clinical symptoms. Schizophr Bull 1999;25:505–17.
56. Nolan K, Volavka J, Czobor P, et al. Aggression and psychopathology in treatment-resistant inpatients with schizophrenia and schizoaffective disorder. J Psychiatr Res 2005;39:109–15.
57. McNiel D, Binder R. The relationship between acute psychiatric symptoms, diagnosis, and short-term risk of violence. Hosp Community Psychiatry 1994;45:133–7.
58. Lanza M, Kayne H, Pattison I, et al. The relationship of behavioral cues to assaultive behavior. Clin Nurs Res 1996;5:6–27.
59. Whittington R, Patterson P. Verbal and non-verbal behavior immediately prior to aggression by mentally disordered people: enhancing the assessment of risk. J Psychiatr Ment Health Nurs 1996;3:47–54.
60. Beauford J, McNiel D, Binder R. Utility of the initial therapeutic alliance in evaluating psychiatric patients' risk of violence. Am J Psychiatry 1997;154:1272–6.
61. Steinert T. Prediction of inpatient violence. Acta Psychiatr Scand Suppl 2002;412:133–41.
62. Binder R, McNiel D. Effects of diagnosis and context on dangerousness. Am J Psychiatry 1988;145:728–32.
63. Lehmann L, McCormick R, Kizer K. A survey of assaultive behavior in Veterans Health Administration facilities. Psychiatr Serv 1999;50:384–9.
64. Miller R, Zadolinnyj K, Hafnew R. Profiles and predictors of assaultiveness for different psychiatric ward populations. Am J Psychiatry 1993;150:1368–73.
65. Tardiff K, Sweillam A. Assaultive behavior among chronic inpatients. Am J Psychiatry 1982;139:212–5.

66. Hill D, Rogers R, Bickford M. Predicting aggressive and socially disruptive behavior in a maximum-security forensic psychiatric hospital. J Forensic Sci 1996;41:56–9.
67. Barratt E, Stanford M, Felthous A, et al. The effects of phenytoin on impulsive and pre-meditated aggression: a controlled study. J Clin Psychopharmacol 1997;17:341–9.
68. Krakowski M, Czobor P. Violence in psychiatric patients: the role of psychosis, frontal lobe impairment, and ward turmoil. Compr Psychiatry 1997;38:230–6.
69. Krakowski M, Convit A, Jaeger J, et al. Neurological impairment in violent schizophrenic inpatients. Am J Psychiatry 1989;146:849–53.
70. Resnick, P. (2016). Risk Assessment for Violence. American Psychiatric Association Annual Meeting. Atlanta, May 16, 2016.
71. Whittington R, Wykes T. Aversive stimulation by staff and violence by psychiatric patients. Br J Clin Psychol 1996;35:11–20.
72. Hodgins S. Mental disorder, intellectual deficiency, and crime: evidence from a birth cohort. Arch Gen Psychiatry 1992;49:475–83.
73. Appelbaum K, Appelbaum P. A model hospital policy on prosecuting patients for presumptively criminal acts. Hosp Community Psychiatry 1991;42:1233–7.
74. Coyne A. Should patients who assault staff be prosecuted? J Psychiatr Ment Health Nurs 2002;9:139–45.
75. Miller R, Maier G. Factors affecting the decision to prosecute mental patients for criminal behavior. Hosp Community Psychiatry 1987;38:50–5.
76. Tarasoff V. Regents of the University of California, 551 P2d 334, 131 Cal. Rptr. 14 (1976).
77. Youngberg V. Romeo, 102 S. Ct. 2452(1982).
78. Dinwiddie W, Briska W. Prosecution of violent psychiatric inpatients: theoretical and practical issues. Int J Law Psychiatry 2004;27:17–29.
79. Hoge S, Gutheil T. The prosecution of psychiatric patients for assaults on staff; a preliminary empirical study. Hosp Community Psychiatry 1987;38:44–9.
80. Ulrich R, Simons R, Losito B, et al. Stress recovery during exposure to natural and urban environments. J Environ Psychol 1991;11:201–30.
81. Ulrich R, Zhu X, Lu Z. Effects of the physical environment of mental health facilities on patient aggression: implications for facility design. Montreal (Canada): Douglas Institute Renewal Project; 2008.
82. Baum A, Valins S. Architectural mediation of residential density and control: crowding and the regulation of social contact. Advances in Experimental Social Psychology, Vol. 12. New York: Academic Press; 1979. p. 131–75.
83. Cox V, Paulus P, McCain G. Prison crowding research: The relevance for prison housing standards and a general approach regarding crowding phenomena. Am Psychol 1984;39(10):1148–59.
84. Ruback R, Carr T, Hopper C. Perceived control in prison: its relation to reporte crowding stress, stress, and symptoms. J Appl Soc Psychol 1986;16(5):375–86.
85. Baillie J. Designing tomorrow's high secure units. Health Estate J 2011;65(6):41–5.
86. Ulrich, R., Begren, L., Lundin, S. Toward a design theory for reducing aggression in psychiatric facilities. Architecture, Research, Care, Health Conference. 2012.
87. Mural J. What's the best nurses' station design for psychiatric hospitals? Healthcare Design 2015.
88. Schoenfisch A, Pompeii L. Weapons use among hospital security personnel. Report to the International Healthcare Security and Safety Foundation 2014.
89. Rosenthal E. When the hospital fires the bullet. The New York Times 2016.
90. Ellison A. The number of armed security guards in hospitals is growing—so is the debate over their necessity. Becker's Hospital Review 2016.

Neuroimaging and Violence

Delaney Smith, MD[a,b],*, Riley Smith, MD[c], Douglas Misquitta, MD[a]

KEYWORDS

- Violence • Neuroimaging • Frontal cortex • Amygdala • Psychopathy
- Antisocial personality disorder

KEY POINTS

- Advancements in the field of neuroimaging have allowed for a greater understanding of the role brain structure and function plays in violence.
- Damage to the prefrontal cortex has long been known to be associated with personality changes, including aggressive tendencies. More recently, it has become clear that there are many substructures in these regions involved in emotional state and social control, with the orbitofrontal cortex being of particular importance in suppressing violent behaviors.
- The limbic system is composed of numerous structures that play an important role in emotional response and regulation. Dysfunction in the amygdala, along with other parts of the limbic system, has been implicated in violence by impairing the brain's ability to interpret threat cues.
- Future directions for neuroimaging may include informing neurobiological models of known treatments and discovery of novel treatment options for violence and associated impulsivity and aggression.

INTRODUCTION

The nineteenth century case of Phineas Gage provides a famous example of brain injury and resultant changes in behavior and personality.[1] Mr Gage was reportedly a mild-mannered individual before he suffered severe injuries to the frontal lobes of his brain in a railroading accident. After the accident, many reports describe him as a very different individual: short-tempered, obnoxious, irresponsible, and violent. Altered personality and behavioral changes can, and have, resulted from trauma/damage to

None of the authors have any disclosures of financial interests or conflicts of interest of any kind.

[a] Department of Psychiatry and Behavioral Health, Ohio State University Wexner Medical Center, 1670 Upham Drive, Suite 130, Columbus, OH 43214, USA; [b] Twin Valley Behavioral Healthcare, 2200 West Broad Street, Columbus, OH 43223, USA; [c] Department of Physical Medicine and Rehabilitation, Wayne State University/Beaumont, 18181 Oakwood Boulevard, Suite 411, Dearborn, MI 48124, USA
* Corresponding author. Twin Valley Behavioral Healthcare, 2200 West Broad Street, Columbus, OH 43223.
E-mail address: Delaney.smith@mha.ohio.gov

the brain, dementia and other neurologic conditions, substance use, and infections. Depending on the part of the brain involved, the resulting changes can include violence, sexually inappropriate behavior, impulsivity, and paranoia. Similarly, certain neuropsychiatric conditions have been associated with abnormal brain architecture, which in turn is believed to contribute to risk or development of disease. Research efforts to understand these changes have considered biological bases and used genetic and adoption studies to explore the contribution of genes, social factors, and environmental factors. There have been studies of neurotransmitter abnormalities, such as reduced serotonin activity.[2] With the past few decades' expansion of neuroimaging techniques, the field has seen a dramatic increase in understanding of the relationship of brain activity and structure to behavioral and clinical findings. One major area of interest has been understanding the brain regions that may contribute to violence.

Violence as a construct has been measured in differing ways across studies. In the articles reviewed, some investigators chose to use a history of interpersonal physical aggression as synonymous with a history of violence. However, even among these studies, there was a difference in approach to accepting self-reported history versus actual legal charges for violent crimes.[3,4] Many studies that were chosen for review instead used diagnoses strongly associated with violence to determine their study and control groups. Psychopathy is one personality construct that has been used in such a way due to its strong association with violence.[5] Psychopaths are typically considered to lack an ability to feel empathy, impairing their judgment and leading to behavior that disregards the well-being of others.[6] Antisocial personality disorder (APD), with its associated hostility, callousness, and impulsivity, also has been used to distinguish between groups when looking at violence markers.[7] Both of these conditions have the benefit of validated measures, such as the Psychopathy Checklist-Revised (PCL-R) and the Personality Assessment Inventory.[5,8] This allows for testing of the theoretic links between brain dysfunction and processing of emotional inputs.[9,10]

Normal behavioral control is influenced by an interplay of multiple processes. Empathy, understanding of consequences, emotional control, and fear are all important components of regulation at a conceptual level.[11] These processes span a wide range of neurologic structures throughout different areas of the brain. Violent behavior is associated with a breakdown in the balance in output and function in the involved structures, some of which are inhibitory and others are excitatory. An understanding of violence and neuroanatomy is difficult without an understanding of normal processes; however, this is complicated, as many of the studies laid out the function of these areas by examining the effects in patients with damage to these areas. In fact, some structures seem to have self-contradictory functions that make simple classification difficult. Although early studies looking at imaging correlates of violence focused on areas known to play a role in emotion, such as the frontal cortex and amygdala, more recent studies have reviewed the entire brain and found other unexpected areas of association.[12,13]

Traumatic and other location-specific brain injuries can give helpful insight into the functioning of specific violence-mediating brain areas. Jorge and Arciniegas[14] found that risk of affective disorders following a traumatic brain injury (TBI) was influenced by many factors, including genetic and psychosocial factors. Similarly, the findings of neuroimaging must be taken in contexts of the entirety of the individual's background and experiences. Specifically looking at those who have had a TBI, not only are preexisting conditions and structures a factor, so too are the changes in life stressors that can occur as a result of the injury itself.[14] Decreased social support, loss of vocational identity, and financial challenges can all exacerbate the actual neurobiological changes that can be seen on imagining.

Aggression and violence in the context of posttraumatic stress disorder (PTSD) also must be considered as a possible confounding factor when looking for imaging changes as a result of trauma.

BRAIN IMAGING TECHNIQUES

Computed tomography (CT) and MRI are the most common ways of imaging the brain. A head CT scan is easy to perform, taking only a few minutes and providing fairly high resolution and sensitivity for certain processes. It uses a focused beam of X-rays passing through the brain at various angles, producing images giving a cross-sectional view of the brain. The head CT can be used for assessment of psychiatric patients who exhibit clinical features that are in some way atypical, such as late-onset depression or psychosis. Head CTs are useful for screening for vascular disease, demyelinating disease, subdural hematomas, and subarachnoid hemorrhages. Limitations include radiation exposure and difficulty visualizing deep brain structures due to the surrounding bony structures.

MRI is more sensitive than CT, and is more likely to detect vascular disease and demyelinating disease. It is also useful in detecting mild neurodegenerative changes, such as in degenerative dementias. MRIs take approximately 45 minutes to perform and are at least twice as expensive as CTs. MRI uses nuclear magnetic resonance causing hydrogen nuclei in the body to release energy at detectable radiofrequencies that are not harmful. MRI provides superior visualization of brain tissue, including deep brain structures, compared with CT.

Brain functioning also can be studied with PET, single-photon emission CT (SPECT), or functional MRI (fMRI). PET is a nuclear medical imaging technique that produces a 3-dimensional image or map of functional processes in the body. SPECT is a nuclear, tomographic imaging technique that allows for study of perfusion in the brain, either in a resting state or during an active task. Indirect measurement of brain activity can be obtained with fMRI by using hemodynamic response.

FRONTAL LOBE AND PREFRONTAL CORTEX

Numerous studies have indicated a link between damage or dysfunction of the frontal lobe, or the prefrontal cortex, and violent, antisocial behavior. Browser and Price[15] indicated, after a 2001 literature review, that there was an association between clinically significant frontal lobe dysfunction and a lack of aggression control. They found this to result in cases of both trauma and neurodegenerative disorders, especially with involvement of the prefrontal cortex. Many studies look at specific regions of the frontal lobe and prefrontal cortex to detect abnormalities associated with violence. Case reports over the past 2 centuries have provided examples of damage to the frontal lobe of the brain and development of symptoms such as poor impulse control, aggression, inappropriate sexual behavior, socially inappropriate conduct, poor judgment, and poor assessment of future consequences. Numerous studies, reviews, and meta-analyses have used neuroimaging to examine and explore the result of damage to these areas of the brain (**Table 1**).

Orbitofrontal Cortex

The orbitofrontal cortex (OFC) is a region of the prefrontal cortex in the frontal lobes that has been associated with decision making and behavioral control.[24,25] Although the prefrontal cortex can be subdivided into many smaller areas, there are marked distinctions between 2 structures that lead to a use of a simple 2-part schema. The dorsolateral area of the prefrontal cortex plays a significant role in cognition, whereas the

Table 1
The results of damage to certain areas of the brain found by using neuroimaging

Modality	Findings	
MRI	Those with antisocial personality disorder had more violent crimes and reduced *prefrontal* gray matter when compared with substance-dependent, psychiatric, and healthy control groups.	Raine et al,[16] 2000
SPECT	Those with alcohol dependence and antisocial personality disorder had greater hypoperfusion of the *frontal lobe* than those with alcohol dependence alone.	Kuruoglu et al,[17] 1996
SPECT	Decreased *prefrontal* activity in adolescents and adults who had attacked others or destroyed property.	Amen et al,[18] 1996
SPECT	Patients with dementia and aggression had significant hypoperfusion of the *bilateral superior frontal lobes* (and of the *left anterior temporal*).	Hirono et al,[19] 2000
PET	Forensic psychiatric patients with violent behavior had decreased *frontal cortical* blood flow or metabolism compared with controls.	Volkow & Tancredi,[20] 1987; Volkow et al,[21] 1995
PET	41 individuals charged with murder or manslaughter had significant *bilateral prefrontal* metabolic decreases compared with controls.	Raine et al,[22] 1997
CT	Veterans with *frontal lobe* injury had more violent behavior compared with those with nonfrontal lobe head injury.	Grafman et al,[23] 1996

Abbreviations: CT, computed tomography; SPECT, single-photon emission computed tomography.

orbitofrontal area is key for emotional and social behavior.[26] This control of social behavior is likely due to integration of emotional and cognitive inputs that the orbitofrontal cortex receives. It has copious reciprocal connections with the amygdala and other limbic structures, as well as the frontal and prefrontal cortex. The somatic marker hypothesis describes this integration and puts forward the idea that the OFC is where decision making is influenced by emotional states.[27] Further integration is done where emotion effects reward-related behavior and leads to suppression of negative emotions in situations in which negative consequences have been learned.[28] This suppression of negative emotions leads to controlled behavior in otherwise angering situations. Functional MRI studies have shown that the orbitofrontal cortex is highly activated while suppressing violent and aggressive feelings.[23] Volumetric studies tie smaller OFC volumes with levels of aggression.[29]

Trauma to these areas of the frontal lobe has been associated with antisocial behavior in the Vietnam Head Injury Study (VHIS), which involved war veterans with head injuries.[23] Veterans with frontal lobe injury showed more aggressive and violent behavior when compared with those with non–frontal lobe head injury. Specifically, 14% of patients with frontal lobe injury engaged in fights or damage of property compared with 4% in those without head injury. In the VHIS study, CT imaging was used to identify injury to the focal mediofrontal and orbitofrontal brain, and found significant association between these areas and increased aggression.

Gansler and colleagues[29] studied 84 male and female patients with diagnoses (using DSM-IV criteria) that included schizophrenia, schizoaffective disorder, bipolar disorder, unipolar affective disorders, anxiety disorders, attention-deficit/hyperactivity disorder, and alcoholism. They found a systematic association of aggression and the left OFC in all patient groups except the participants with bipolar disorder. There was also no OFC-aggression relationship found in the control group. They found reduction of left OFC volume to be a significant substrate for aggression, and they suggested a role for the left OFC in emotional and/or instrumental types of aggression.

Anterior Cingulate Cortex

The anterior cingulate cortex (ACC) is often divided into dorsal and ventral segments and has connections to the prefrontal cortex, parietal cortex, and frontal eye fields.[30] The dorsal ACC has functions primarily concerning cognition. The ventral component has connections to the limbic system, including the amygdala, nucleus accumbens, and insular cortex. Some researchers dismiss the anatomic division and state that all functions are carried out by both portions.[31] The ACC has been noted to have an abundance of spindle cells, which seem to be found in only humans and other animals with notable intelligence (apes, cetaceans, elephants). The ACC plays a role in error detection, as well as in integration of conflicting inputs (eg, the Stroop Task). There is additional activity in the ACC during tests with monetary rewards and losses depending on the correct answer. It is involved in acts of self-control, perseverance, and delayed tasks.[32,33] It also plays a role in appraising stimuli that induces fear and anxiety so as to regulate the autonomic response and thereby modulate fear expression.[34] The ACC is also thought to play a role in empathy and is activated in a similar manner when exposed to a disgusting odor as when shown a video with a facial expression of disgust.[35] The ACC may be part of the interpretation of mental states of others and outflow to emotional centers that form the basis of empathy.[36,37] When anger is induced in healthy men, there is increased activity of the ventral anterior cingulate cortex.[38] There was also increased activation when male subjects were asked to suppress sexual arousal, indicating the ACC plays a role in emotional regulation.[39]

A 2009 meta-analysis of 43 independent studies also demonstrated significant association between antisocial behavior and reduced structure and function of the prefrontal brain, specifically the right OFC, right ACC, and left dorsolateral prefrontal cortex (DLPFC), a functional structure associated to the OFC.[40] Their findings pointed to antisocial behavior being associated more with right-sided prefrontal pathology. For example, several studies involving patients with antisocial or psychopathic features had shown that patients with damage to the right OFC had impaired social conduct, decision making, and emotional processing.[27,41–43] In comparison, those with lesions to the left OFC had normal social and interpersonal behavior. Similarly, studies by Danckert and colleagues[44] and Hornak and colleagues[45] found that unilateral lesions to the right ACC were associated with impairment in inhibitory control and emotional processing, whereas lesions to the left ACC were not.

On the other hand, damage to the left DLPFC in particular has been associated with impairment in attention, cognitive flexibility, impulse control, and other processes associated with higher cognition and self-regulation.[46–48] Yang and Raine,[40] when considering these results, suggested that reduction in the right prefrontal cortex (OFC, ACC) was associated with emotional deficits and poor decision making in antisocial individuals, whereas reduction in the left DLPFC was linked more with features of impulsivity and poor behavioral control. Psychopathic individuals have been shown to make more errors in cues presented by their right visual field, which involves initial processing by the left hemisphere of the brain. Kosson,[49] in 1998, proposed that psychopathic individuals may have problems with attention due to difficulty in processing information in the left hemisphere, and difficulty in shifting attention from the left to the right hemisphere. Thus, it may be that damage to left-sided areas of the brain, such as the DLPFC, negatively impacts attention. Yang and Raine[40] suggested that right-sided deficits to the OFC and ACC may indirectly worsen attention, as these regions play a key role in processing secondary cues, such as emotional content, and therefore might lead to less effective direction of attention to important information in the right hemisphere when needed. In the studies reviewed in this meta-analysis, fMRI was found to have the best ability to detect brain activity changes associated with antisocial behavior.[40,50,51]

Insular Cortex

Also known as the insula, the insular cortex lies deep within the lateral sulcus. It has been linked to a wide range of functions, including homeostasis, emotions, consciousness, self-awareness, and interpersonal experience. It can be divided into an anterior and a posterior portion. The anterior receives information from the thalamus and there are reciprocal projections to the amygdala. The posterior insula is connected by afferents and efferents to the secondary somatosensory cortex, as well as the thalamus. The insula is involved in the generation of a response of disgust, both to putrid smells as well as images or thoughts of contamination.[35,52–54] The similar response to imagined and experienced stimuli indicates the insula plays a role in creating an internalization of stimuli. It has been proposed that this response may be the source of emotional experience as a result of bodily states and autonomic responses. It also plays a role in identifying violation of norms, fear, and uncertainty.[55,56] The insula is often considered to be a structure of the limbic system that developed early and maintains conserved functions. Despite this, the insula contains a high density of spindle cells that are present only in great apes, humans, and a few other species. These cells have been associated with integration and processing of contradictory information and new learning. The insula may be a site of cognitive and emotional integration that leads to empathy and self-awareness.[57] Empathy and self-awareness may be a result of integrating homeostatic and imagined stimuli into conscious states.[58]

Several studies have highlighted decreased glucose metabolism in the prefrontal and orbitofrontal cortex in association with violence and aggression. For example, Goyer and colleagues[59] used PET to examine regional cerebral metabolic rates of glucose metabolism (rCMRG) in the frontal lobes, and reported a significant relationship between impulsive aggression and frontal cortical functioning, based on a negative correlation between history of aggressive impulse difficulties and rCMRG. Raine and colleagues[60] reported selected reduction in prefrontal rCMRG when comparing murderers with an age-matched and sex-matched healthy control sample. Raine and colleagues[22] also used PET scans during continuous performance tasks by offenders charged with murder, with the scans showing significantly reduced glucose metabolism in the medial and lateral prefrontal cortex compared with the control group. They concluded, based on further study, that lower glucose metabolism created a greater predisposition to violence, as they found that murders without any clear history of psychosocial deficits had significantly lower glucose metabolism compared with murderers who did have an early psychosocial deprivation.[22,60,61]

Antisocial subjects showed activation deficit in the left frontal gyrus (and other brain areas) when compared with healthy controls in an investigation looking at working memory.[62] Subtle working memory deficits were seen in the schizophrenia without a history of violence group and in the antisocial personality group. Severe deficits were seen in the individuals with schizophrenia with a serious physical violence history relative to the healthy group. This group had activation deficit bilaterally in the frontal lobe and precuneus compared with the healthy group, and in the right inferior parietal region when compared with the individuals with schizophrenia without a history of violence during the working memory load condition. Frontal bilateral activity was negatively associated with ratings of violence across all patients with schizophrenia. Patients with APD, compared with healthy controls, showed activation deficit in the left frontal gyrus, anterior cingulate, and precuneus. This reduced functional response in the frontal and parietal regions leads to serious violence in schizophrenia, perhaps via impaired executive functioning.

Joyal and colleagues[63] also saw decreased frontal activation in schizophrenic patients with APD and substance abuse. Activation was significantly less in the frontal basal cortices during go/no-go tasks compared with those solely with schizophrenia, as well as nonviolent persons without a mental illness. The regions that showed significantly higher activation were the frontal motor, premotor, and anterior cingulate regions in the group with schizophrenia, APD, and substance use disorder compared with schizophrenia alone. Smith[64] suggested disinhibition in psychopathic individuals may be related to deficits in processing information in the left dorsolateral prefrontal brain based on attenuated activation in that brain region during performance of response inhibition tasks when compared with healthy controls. Kiehl,[65] in an fMRI study, reported an unusual pattern of activation of the prefrontal (and limbic) region in psychopathic individuals when compared with controls in the processing of emotional words.

Volumetric studies also have demonstrated structural differences in the frontal and prefrontal areas of the brain that may contribute to violence. Dolan[66] conducted a quantitative MRI study (1998) in which he found reduced prefrontal brain volumes in aggressive offenders with APD compared with healthy controls. Dolan[67] concluded that subtle structural and functional deficits in the neural circuits of the frontal and tempero-limbic brain involved in impulse control and emotional information processing were present in those with psychopathic and antisocial behaviors. MRIs have been used to measure and compare the volume of gray and white matter in the frontal lobes in individuals with APD and in a control group. In comparison with the controls, they found that the APD group had a significant reduction in prefrontal gray matter.[16,68]

Tiihonen and colleagues[69] used voxel-based morphometry of the gray matter to compare 26 violent offenders with 25 healthy men, and found numerous focal, bilateral areas of atrophy in the brain, including in the frontopolar cortex (superior and medial frontal gyrus) and orbitofrontal gyrus. Violent offenders, when compared with healthy men, also had decreased white matter density in the right medial frontal gyrus. The findings of Tiihonen and colleagues[69] support hypotheses that the frontal cortex and orbitofrontal cortex, key areas in regulation of violent and aggressive behavior, are malfunctioning in persistently violent offenders with histories of early-onset stable antisocial behavior, and that offenders with psychopathy have difficulties in neuropsychological tasks that depend on the orbitofrontal cortex.

Narayan and colleagues[70] used MRI to explore the correlation between violence and brain structure in APD and schizophrenia. Violence was associated with cortical thinning in the medial inferior frontal and lateral sensory motor cortex, particularly in the right hemisphere, and surrounding association areas (Brodmann areas 10, 11, 12, and 32). These data have been used to support the hypothesis that somatic states are essential to the decision-making process, and that impairs the ability to weigh potential consequences of actions and in these individuals may lead to aggression.[71]

THE LIMBIC SYSTEM

The limbic system is composed of a key group of structures in emotional response and regulation. The grouping is primary historical and based on the structures separating, or creating a border between, the cerebral hemispheres and the brainstem.[72] Because the structures that are attributed to the limbic system are similar only in their location, they display a very broad range of functions, including emotion, behavior, motivation, long-term memory, olfaction, and awareness of somatic stimuli. From its origin as a border region, it was realized that this system was pivotal in emotional response. For example, early fMRI studies showed that criminals with psychopathy had less affect-related activity in limbic structures compared with their nonpsychopathic criminal counterparts.[73] Various cortical, subcortical, and diencephalon structures have been included as part of the limbic system having been linked to emotion (**Box 1**). Because the limbic system is a collection of functionally related structures, there is controversy regarding what structures should be included and whether it is an obsolete concept.[74]

Amygdala

The amygdala are the neural structures most directly related to fear response through direct and indirect studies.[75,76] Direct electric stimulation to the amygdala has been shown to result in a repeatable immediate fear state. There are 3 principal divisions of the amygdala: the basolateral nucleus, central nucleus, and corticomedial nuclei.[77] Further subdivision is possible, with the basolateral nucleus containing basal, lateral, and accessory basal nuclei; and the corticomedial subdividing into the cortical and medial nuclei.[78]

Projections from association cortical areas as well as high-order sensory cortex reach the basolateral nucleus and project onto the cingulate gyrus, dorsomedial thalamic nuclei, hippocampus, and orbitofrontal cortex, as well as the central nucleus of the amygdala.[79] In addition to receiving input from the basolateral nuclei, the central nuclei also receive input from the viscerosensory structures of the brain stem and give off efferent fibers to the autonomic nuclei and hypothalamus.[80] The corticomedial

---

Box 1
Structures of the limbic system

Cortical Areas

Limbic lobe

Orbitofrontal cortex

Piriform cortex

Entorhinal cortex

Hippocampus

Fornix

Subcortical Areas

Septal nuclei

Amygdala

Nucleus accumbens

Diencephalic Areas

Hypothalamus

Mammillary bodies

Anterior nuclei of thalamus

nuclei receive projections from the olfactory bulb and cortex.[81] The basolateral nuclei play a key role in attaching conscious significance to a stimulus and integrating the emotional response into memory. The basolateral nuclei play a role in the potentiation of the autonomic system's response to emotionally charged stimuli.

As stated previously, electric stimulation of the amygdala can lead to immediate fear. However, stimulation to the hippocampus leads to activation of the amygdala and in turn a delayed fear response after the discharges have reached the amygdala. There is additionally a functional difference between the left and right amygdala. It has been shown that stimulation of the right amygdala induces primarily fear and sadness, whereas stimulation of the left amygdala could result in emotions neither negative (fear, anxiety, sadness) nor positive (happiness).[75] It is thought the right amygdala self-monitors for emotional stimulus, whereas the left processes consciousness and language.[82,83] There are additional sex-based differences in the relative size of the right versus the left amygdala, with men tending to have a larger right amygdala and women having a larger left amygdala.[84]

The amygdala has an additional key role in the formation of memory and tying memory to emotional events. As a result, the amygdala plays a key role in fear conditioning.[85] There also have been volumetric studies that correlate size of the amygdala with the extent of an individual social network, a person's ability to interpret social information from other persons' faces, and possibly to a person's emotional intelligence.[86,87]

The amygdala has long been identified as a structure of interest in individuals with disorders commonly associated with violence. It has been hypothesized that dysfunction in the amygdala and other parts of the limbic system contributes to difficulty interpreting threat cues, such that there is increased aggression in these individuals.[88] A longitudinal study reviewed adult men with a history of aggression and future risk for aggression based on amygdala volume measured by MRI.[89] When looking at the historical data, the investigators found lower right amygdala volume was associated with increased proactive aggression and adolescent psychopathic features, whereas left amygdala volume reduction was associated with increased teacher-reported aggression and callousness. Concurrent psychological testing showed a decrease in bilateral amygdala volume was associated with higher premeditated aggression by self-report on the aggression subscale of the Adult Self-Report and Premeditated Aggression Scale. A unique function of this study included a review of postscan outcomes that showed that reduced bilateral amygdala volume also was associated with an increase in future risk of committing violence, higher verbal and physical aggression, and increase in follow-up psychopathy on the Self-Report of Psychopathy-III short form.

In the past 10 years, models of amygdala function have been put forth to try to account for inconsistency in some of the earlier research. One such model differentiated between functioning of the basolateral amygdala (BLA), an inhibitory nucleus, and the central amygdala (CA), which is regarded as a key component in stress reactions.[90,91] MRIs of male violent offenders with psychopathy have shown reduction in BLA tissue volumes and increased volume in CA when compared with controls.[12]

Recent imaging research by Yoder and colleagues[92] helps to clarify the role of differing subnuclei in the amygdala through fMRI processing to isolate violence-specific neural activity. They found that elevated self-centered impulsivity scores on the Psychopathic Personality Inventory-Revised (PPI-R) were associated with decreased coupling between the BLA and ventrolateral prefrontal cortex, and that Fearless Dominance scores were associated with increased coupling between the CA and posterior insula.[92] This work supports the key concept that the amygdala does not function as one unitary structure, but instead that the unique functional components of the complex separately mediate violence-related behavioral responses.

Basal Ganglia and Nucleus Accumbens

The basal ganglia is a deep brain circuit made up of a network of 7 nuclei that are involved in motor planning, reward-based learning, and action selection and gating, among other functions.[93] Basal ganglia dysfunction has been implicated in numerous neuropsychiatric disorders, including Wilson disease, schizophrenia, Parkinson disease, and Huntington chorea. The nucleus accumbens is a component of the basal ganglia and together with the olfactory tubercle, they form the ventral striatum. The nucleus accumbens is composed of 2 structures: the nucleus accumbens core and the nucleus accumbens shell. These areas have different neuron morphologies and different function. Both portions of the nucleus accumbens play a role in aversion, including fear, impulsivity, motivation, pleasure seeking, and reinforcement learning.[94] Because of its connections to pleasure seeking and reinforcement, it plays a key role in addiction.[95]

The nucleus accumbens receives inputs from the BLA, prefrontal cortex, and the ventral tegmental area. It distributes outputs to the basal ganglia, and indirectly to the orbitofrontal cortex, thalamus, striatum, substantia nigra, and reticular formation.[96] Because it receives significant input from the amygdala and has output to the orbitofrontal cortex, the nucleus accumbens is thought to play a key role in regulation of behavior.[97] It also has been implicated in reversal learning. This is the process of overwriting previous knowledge when new sensory and cognitive information is presented. It allows individuals to alter their values and goals when the individual faces new consequences, that is, learns from experience.[97] An MRI study demonstrated a reduction of nucleus accumbens volume in individuals with elevated psychopathy scores on the PCL-R, which the investigators felt represented differing interpretations of cost-benefit evaluations that might lead to pathologic conclusions.[97] One can then see how such faulty outcome assessments could lead to behaviors, such as predatory aggression, that do not fit into the typical societal expectations and are often counterproductive to the goals of the individual undertaking the behavior.

The shell of the nucleus accumbens acts in reward perception and is associated with positive reinforcement. It is the primary area of action and learning associated with addictive drugs and addictive behaviors.[98–100] The shell receives significant dopaminergic input and is most directly stimulated by amphetamines and opiates, as well as rewarding experiences.[97] It was the shell of the nucleus accumbens that was stimulated in the classic rat experiment in pleasure. Electrodes were placed into this region of the brain and the septal nuclei (another "pleasure center") of the rat, and were stimulated when the rat pressed a lever. The rats would constantly press the lever to receive this stimulation and would forego food and water, leading to their death.[101] There was also an effect on aversion-related cognition. The core is more directly involved in motor learning associated with reward acquisition.

The dorsal striatum, made up of the caudate nucleus and the putamen, and the ventral striatum serve as the primary inputs to the basal ganglia. Neurons in these areas of the striatum have been identified as helping to process sensory stimuli and use the information to predict reward and code the reward value of actions, and as such are essential for learning.[98] Abnormal caudate nucleus activation has been shown in individuals with schizophrenia by fMRI[3] and structural MRI research has shown larger caudate nucleus volumes to be associated with higher aggression levels in individuals with schizophrenia.[102,103] Similarly, the increased putamen volume associated with APD has been hypothesized to be related to behavioral disinhibition and impulsivity in these individuals.[104]

Thalamus

One case report of a woman with a resolution of dementia-related aggression following an infarct of the anterior thalamic nucleus (ATN) sheds light on another possible brain region involved in violence.[105] The investigators felt that this response was due to the important connection the ATN represents between the temporal and frontal lobes, both of which are strongly implicated in aggression. A possible role of the thalamus is further supported by a 2013 study that found reduced thalamic volumes in individuals with a history of serious violence and psychosocial deprivation.[106] The brain changes may represent abnormal development of this important region as a result of this deprivation, which may later predispose one toward aggression. Barkataki and his group[3] also have studied the role of the thalamus in mediating violence and identified decreased activation in a subgroup of people with schizophrenia who had a history of violence compared with those who did not. They concluded that when the thalamus is not properly fulfilling its role in filtering out unnecessary information, an individual is more susceptible to overstimulation, which could lead to a lack of controlling violence.

Hippocampus

Studies that have reviewed brain structure in those individuals with schizophrenia who have engaged in violence have demonstrated changes in the hippocampus and associated structures. Barkataki and colleagues[3] undertook a study to try to clarify these relationships. Brain MRIs were performed on men with APD, men with schizophrenia with a history of violence, and men with schizophrenia without violence, and a control group of men without violence, schizophrenia, or APD. They found that the group with both schizophrenia and a history of violence had a reduction in their hippocampal volume and the brain as a whole. Similarly, a 2010 study in a Chinese sample found structural differences between those with schizophrenia who had been found guilty of murder and others.[51] When compared with healthy controls, murderers with schizophrenia had reduced gray matter volume in the hippocampal and parahippocampal gyrus, whereas those who had committed murder but did not have schizophrenia had only a reduction in the parahippocampal gyrus. While not looking specifically at murder, Kumari and colleagues[4] found that individuals with schizophrenia and a history of severe violence as tested on the Gunn and Robertson Scale had a reduction in the hippocampal volume that was not seen in those without violence. This finding also has been shown in adolescents, with those who were incarcerated for committing homicide having reduced gray matter volumes in the hippocampus in addition to the posterior insula on MRI when compared with incarcerated juveniles who had not committed homicide.[107]

CEREBELLUM

As methods for identifying brain structure and function have improved, neuroimaging studies have been performed globally instead of focusing on areas with preexistent hypotheses regarding their likely relationship to violence and aggression. These studies have revealed several other areas of potential interest in the brain.

In an MRI volumetry study comparing violent offenders with APD with matched controls, the offender group was found to have larger right cerebellar gray matter and left cerebellar white matter.[69] The effect size increased when looking at the subgroup of offenders who also scored high for psychopathy on the PCL-R. The investigators interpreted the increased brain volumes in these regions to represent neurodevelopmental changes consistent with the development of APD. An evaluation of voxel-based morphometry of MRI scans of individuals with schizophrenia who have committed serious violent offenses compared with a nonoffender schizophrenia group also revealed changes in cerebellar volume between the groups that was believed to be related to impaired verbal working memory, which is essential for cognition.[108]

TEMPORAL, OCCIPITAL, AND PARIETAL REGIONS

The brain's temporal region has been identified as a potential region of interest in several large studies.[98,109] The role of the anterior temporal cortex, along with areas of the prefrontal cortex, in assessing active information in comparison with stored social information has been thought to contribute to empathy and moral reasoning and, thus, when impaired, to predispose toward aggressive responses.[110] A case report from Canada described an individual who had severe aggressive episodes associated with interictal temporal epileptiform activity.[111] A study looking at individuals with Down syndrome who had no aggressive tendencies, and in fact often fail to recognize aggressive cues in others, demonstrated a decreased activation of the medial temporal structures in response to threats, further supporting the idea that this area is important in understanding and responding to social situations and mediating aggressive responses.[112]

Violent offenders have been observed to have increased occipital white matter when compared with healthy subjects.[69] The investigators of this study found similarities between the brain region changes in methamphetamine users observed in other studies, but concluded that rather than a neurotoxic effect of the drug, these changes might represent genetic, environmental, or other factors that increased the likelihood to use drugs.[113] Bertsch and colleagues[114] found reduced gray matter volumes in the occipital region in offenders with APD who scored high on psychopathic personality traits. Bilateral parietal white matter volumes are larger in violent offenders diagnosed with psychopathy.[69]

SUMMARY

Brain imaging cannot yet identify thoughts or motives. Its role, traditionally, has been to aid in diagnosis and assessment, and has been only one element of a larger clinical examination that also involves comprehensive history taking (psychiatric, medical, family, legal, and social histories); collateral information; laboratory testing; neurologic and psychiatric mental status examinations; and, as needed, neuropsychological testing. The most likely use of imaging in the short term may continue to be to support diagnosis, or rule outs of diagnoses, alongside other established ways of identifying clinical signs of the illness. In the long term, the role of imaging may become more broad and multifaceted. As imaging technologies continue to expand, and our own understanding grows, it may provide innovative ways in a variety of contexts of analyzing, interpreting, and understanding human behavior and the neurologic underpinnings of both normal behavior and of symptoms and behavior resulting from brain disease or damage.

One way neuroimaging information about violence and other related impulsive disorders is beginning to be used is to test treatment hypotheses or aid the development of novel treatment approaches. Anticonvulsants, antipsychotics, and serotonergic agents have long been known to have the potential to treat impulsive aggression.[115] With imaging, the actual impact of these agents on brains can be demonstrated through pretreatment and posttreatment studies. One double-blind, placebo-controlled study administered 3 days of the antipsychotic quetiapine and then performed an fMRI to monitor brain connectivity while participants engaged in a violent video game.[116] They found that the quetiapine group had changes in amygdala connectivity that were not seen with the placebo group. Italian physicians were able to use MRI and intraoperative microrecording to determine the precise location for implantation of deep-brain stimulation electrodes into the posterior hypothalamic region bilaterally.[117,118] Their technique resulted in a reduction of aggressive symptoms in 6 of 7 participants.

Neuroscientific methods also may prove helpful in testing and validating neuropsychological tools. As imaging data for those with violent tendencies improves, it can be correlated with clinical findings and results on established personality and diagnostic inventories, and the validity of these tests can be improved. Similarly, tools for the prediction of violence recidivism may be able to be refined by the information gathered from these studies.[119]

Husted and colleagues[115] described a growing trend in criminal trials of neuroimaging studies, such as PET, SPECT, and fMRI, being used by defenses to demonstrate that a defendant has a brain disorder, or at the sentencing phase for purposes of mitigation. They detailed the use of structural MRI results to partially substantiate multiple indicators of brain dysfunction and psychiatric illness as exculpatory evidence by the defense team. The investigators detailed the complexity of using these findings to reflect on the complex decision making and behaviors on the day of the crime, and the difficulty of connecting brain imaging test results with a person's set of cognitions, feelings, and experiences. They concluded that in most cases such information could be considered a mitigating factor to help determine culpability as well as appropriate punishment and/or treatment. Others have considered neuroscience-based credibility assessments as a possible way to aid courts in determining an individual's knowledge of a crime or truthfulness as well as to predict recidivism, although with the caveat that studies need to improve in the future if this is going to come to fruition.[120]

In future studies, more specific categorizing of violent offenders, or of the degree and nature of their impulsivity or violent acts, may be helpful in better clarifying the relationship between the brain and behavior. There is a likely role for consideration, and control, for other known risk factors for violence, particularly socioeconomic deprivation and trauma. Further study also is needed with regard to the impact of substance use on these brain findings to elucidate when substance use disorders are a result of abnormal findings and when they are the cause.

Finally, like with research into the genetics of aggression, consideration also must be given to the ethical issues that may arise if overzealous attempts are made at extrapolating these broader findings to the individual level and used to stigmatize people as presenting a threat to society based solely on neuroimaging findings.[121]

REFERENCES

1. Macmillan M. Phineas Gage–unravelling the myth. Psychologist 2008;21: 828–31.
2. Frankle GW, Lombardo I, New AS, et al. Brain serotonin transporter distribution in subjects with impulsive aggressivity: a positron emission study with [11C] McN 5652. Am J Psychiatry 2005;162(5):915–23.
3. Barkataki I, Kumari V, Das M, et al. Neural correlates of deficient response inhibition in mentally disordered violent individuals. Behav Sci Law 2008;26:51–64.
4. Kumari V, Barkataki I, Goswami S, et al. Dysfunctional, but not functional, impulsivity is associated with a history of seriously violent behaviour and reduced

orbitofrontal and hippocampal volumes in schizophrenia. Psychiatry Res 2009; 173:39–44.

5. Hare RD. The Hare psychopathy checklist-revised. 2nd edition. Toronto: Multi-Health Systems; 2003.

6. Anderson JS, Treiman SM, Ferguson MA, et al. Violence: heightened brain attentional network response is selectively muted in Down syndrome. J Neurodev Disord 2015;7(1):15.

7. American Psychiatric Association. Diagnostic and statistical manual of mental disorders. 5th edition. Arlington (VA): American Psychiatric Publishing; 2013.

8. Walters GD, Diamond PM, Magaletta PR, et al. Taxometric analysis of the antisocial features scale of the personality assessment inventory in federal prison inmates. Assessment 2007;14(4):351–60.

9. Dolan M, Fullman R. Psychopathy and functional magnetic resonance imaging blood oxygenation level-dependent responses to emotional faces in violent patients with schizophrenia. Biol Psychiatry 2009;66:570–7.

10. Dolan M. What imagining tells us about violence in antisocial men. Crim Behav Ment Health 2010;20:199–214.

11. Scarpa A, Raine A. Psychophysiology of anger and violent behavior. Psychiatr Clin North Am 1997;20:375–94.

12. Boccardi M, Frisoni GB, Hare RD. Cortex and amygdala morphology in psychopathy. Psychiatry Res 2011;193(2):85–92.

13. Eichelman B. The limbic system and aggression in humans. Neurosci Biobehav Rev 1983;7(3):391–4.

14. Jorge RE, Arciniegas DB. Mood disorder after TBI. Psychiatr Clin North Am 2014;37(1):13–29.

15. Brower MC, Price BH. Neuropsychiatry of frontal lobe dysfunction in violent and criminal behaviour: a critical review. J Neurol Neurosurg Psychiatry 2001;71: 720–6.

16. Raine A, Lencz T, Bihrle S, et al. Reduced prefrontal gray matter volume and reduced autonomic activity in antisocial personality disorder. Arch Gen Psychiatry 2000;57:119–27 [discussion: 128–9].

17. Kuruoglu AC, Arikan Z, Vural G, et al. Single photon emission computerized tomography in chronic alcoholism. Antisocial personality disorder may be associated with decreased frontal perfusion. Br J Psychiatry 1996;169(3):348–54.

18. Amen DG, Stubblefield M, Carmicheal B, et al. Brain SPECT findings and aggressiveness. Ann Clin Psychiatry 1996;8:129–37.

19. Hirono N, Mega MS, Dinov ID, et al. Left frontotemporal hypoperfusion is associated with aggression in patients with dementia. Arch Neurol 2000;57:861–6.

20. Volkow ND, Tancredi L. Neural substrates of violent behavior: a preliminary study with positron emission tomography. Br J Psychiatry 1987;151:668–73.

21. Volkow ND, Tancredi LR, Grant C, et al. Brain glucose metabolism in violent psychiatric patients: a preliminary study. Psychiatry Res 1995;61:243–53.

22. Raine A, Buchsbaum M, LaCasse L. Brain abnormalities in murderers indicated by positron emission tomography. Biol Psychiatry 1997;42(6):495–508.

23. Grafman J, Schwab K, Warden D, et al. Frontal lobe injuries, violence and aggression: a report of the Vietnam head injury study. Neurology 1996;46: 1231–8.

24. Davidson RJ, Putnam KM, Larson CL. Dysregulation in the neural circuitry of emotion regulation—possible prelude to violence. Science 2000;289:591–4.

25. Weiger WA, Bear DM. An approach to the neurology of aggression. J Psychiatr Res 1988;22:85–98.

26. Fuster JM. Executive frontal functions. Exp Brain Res 2000;133:66–70.
27. Bechara A. The role of emotion in decision making: evidence from neurological patients with orbitofrontal damage. Brain Cogn 2004;55:30–40.
28. Rolls ET. The functions of the orbitofrontal cortex. Neurocase 1999;5:311–2.
29. Gansler DA, McLaughlin NC, Iguchi L, et al. A multivariate approach to aggression and the orbital frontal cortex in psychiatric patients. Psychiatry Res 2009; 171:145–54.
30. Bush G, Luu P, Posner MI. Cognitive and emotional influences in anterior cingulate cortex. Trends Cogn Sci 2000;4:215–22.
31. Heilbronner SR, Hayden BY. Dorsal anterior cingulate cortex: a bottom-up view. Annu Rev Neurosci 2016;14:149–70.
32. Aron AR, Robbins TW, Poldrack RA. Inhibition at the right inferior frontal cortex. Trends Cogn Sci 2004;8:170–7.
33. Picton TW, Stuss DT, Alexander MP, et al. Effects of focal frontal lesions on response inhibition. Cereb Cortex 2007;17:826–38.
34. Milad MR, Quirk GJ, Pitman RK, et al. A role for the human dorsal anterior cingulate cortex in fear expression. Biol Psychiatry 2007;62:1191–4.
35. Wicker B, Keysers C, Plailly J, et al. Both of us disgusted in my insula: the common neural basis of seeing and feeling disgust. Neuron 2003;40:655–64.
36. Decety J, Jackson PL. The functional architecture of human empathy. Behav Cogn Neurosci Rev 2004;3:71–100.
37. DeMartino B, Kumaran D, Seymour B, et al. Frames, biases, and rational decision-making in the human brain. Science 2006;313:684–7.
38. Dougherty DD, Shin LM, Alpert NM, et al. Anger in healthy men: a PET study using script-driven imagery. Biol Psychiatry 1999;46:466–72.
39. Beauregard M, Lévesque J, Bourgouin P. Neural correlates of conscious self-regulation of emotion. J Neurosci 2001;21:RC165.
40. Yang Y, Raine A. Prefrontal structural and functional brain imaging findings in antisocial, violent, and psychopathic individuals: a meta-analysis. Psychiatry Res 2009;174:81–8.
41. Angrilli A, Palomba D, Cantagallo A, et al. Emotional impairment after right orbitofrontal lesion in a patient without cognitive deficits. Neuroreport 1999;10: 1741–6.
42. Arciniegas DB, Wortzel HS. Emotional and behavioral dyscontrol after traumatic brain injury. Psychiatr Clin North Am 2014;37(1):31–53.
43. Eslinger PJ, Damasio AR. Severe disturbance of higher cognition after bilateral frontal lobe ablation: patient EVR. Neurology 1985;35:1731–41.
44. Danckert J, Maruff P, Ymer C, et al. Goal-directed selective attention and response competition monitoring: evidence from unilateral parietal and anterior cingulate lesions. Neuropsychology 2000;14:16–28.
45. Hornak J, Bramham J, Rolls ET, et al. Changes in emotion after circumscribed surgical lesions of the orbitofrontal and cingulate cortices. Brain 2003;126: 1691–712.
46. Grattan LM, Eslinger PJ. Long-term psychological consequences of childhood frontal lobe lesion in patient DT. Brain Cogn 1992;20:185–95.
47. Hornak J, O'Doherty J, Bramham J, et al. Reward-related reversal learning after surgical excisions in orbito-frontal or dorsolateral prefrontal cortex in humans. J Cogn Neurosci 2004;16:463–78.
48. Stuss DT, Floden D, Alexander MP, et al. Stroop performance in focal lesion patients: dissociation of processes and frontal lobe lesion location. Neuropsychologia 2001;39:771–86.

49. Kosson DS. Psychopathy and dual-task performance under focusing conditions. J Abnorm Psychol 1998;105(3):391–400.
50. Yang Y, Raine A, Lencz T, et al. Volume reduction in prefrontal gray matter in unsuccessful criminal psychopaths. Biol Psychiatry 2005;57(10):1103–8.
51. Yang Y, Raine A, Han CB, et al. Reduced hippocampal and parahippocampal volumes in murderers with schizophrenia. Psychiatry Res 2010;182(1):9–13.
52. Jabbi M, Bastiaansen J, Keysers C. A common anterior insula representation of disgust observation, experience and imagination shows divergent functional connectivity pathways. PLoS One 2008;3:e2939.
53. Wehring HJ, Carpenter WT. Violence and schizophrenia. Schizophr Bull 2011; 37(5):877–8.
54. Xue G, Lu Z, Levin IP, et al. The impact of prior risk experiences on subsequent risky decision-making: the role of the insula. Neuroimage 2010;50:709–16.
55. Sanfey AG, Rilling JK, Aronson JA, et al. The neural basis of economic decision-making in the ultimatum game. Science 2003;300:1755–8.
56. Schiffer B, Pawliczek C, Mu Ller B, et al. Neural mechanisms underlying cognitive control of men with lifelong antisocial behavior. Psychiatry Res 2014;222: 43–51.
57. De Martino B, Kumaran D, et al. Frames, biases, and rational decision-making in the human brain. Science 2006;313:684–7.
58. GuiXue G, Lu Z, et al. The impact of prior risk experiences on subsequent risky decision-making: the role of the insula. NeuroImage 2010;50:709–16.
59. Goyer PF, Andreason PJ, Semple WE, et al. Positron-emission tomography and personality disorders. Neuropsychopharmacology 1994;10(1):21–8.
60. Raine A, Buchsbaum MS, Stanley J, et al. Selective reductions in prefrontal glucose metabolism in murderers. Biol Psychiatry 1994;36(6):365–73.
61. Raine A, Meloy JR, Bihrle S, et al. Reduced prefrontal and increased subcortical brain functioning assessed using positron emission tomography in predatory and affective murderers. Behav Sci Law 1998;16:319–32.
62. Kumari V, Aasen I, Taylor P, et al. Neural dysfunction and violence in schizophrenia: an fMRI investigation. Schizophr Res 2006;84(1):144–64.
63. Joyal CC, Putkonen A, Mancini-Marie A, et al. Violent persons with schizophrenia and comorbid disorders: a functional magnetic resonance imaging study. Schizophr Res 2007;91(1–3):97–102.
64. Smith AM. An fMRI investigation of frontal lobe functioning in psychopathy and schizophrenia during a go/no go task. Diss Abstr Int B Sci Eng 2000;61:128.
65. Kiehl KA. A neuroimaging investigation of affective, cognitive and language functions in psychopathy. Diss Abstr Int B Sci 2000;61:2766.
66. Dolan M. Impulsivity/aggression: relationships with 5–HT, neurocognitive function, and structural MRI in personality disordered offenders [PhD thesis]. Manchester (United Kingdom): University of Manchester; 1998.
67. Dolan M. What neuroimaging tells us about psychopathic disorders. Hosp Med 2002;63(6):337–40.
68. Raine A, Ishikawa SS, Arce E, et al. Hippocampal structural asymmetry in unsuccessful psychopaths. Biol Psychiatry 2004;55(2):185–91.
69. Tiihonen J, Rossi R, Laakso MP, et al. Brain anatomy of persistent violent offenders: more rather than less. Psychiatry Res 2008;163:201–12.
70. Narayan VM, Narr KL, Kumari V, et al. Regional cortical thinning in subjects with violent antisocial personality disorder or schizophrenia. Am J Psychiatry 2007; 164(9):1418–27.

71. Domasio AR. The somatic marker hypothesis and the possible functions of the prefrontal cortex. Philos Trans R Soc Lond Biol Sci 1996;351(1346):1413–20.

72. Broca P. Anatomie comparee des circonvolutions cerebrales: le grand lobe limbique et la scissure limbique dans la serie des mammifères. Revue d'Anthropologie 1878;1:385–498.

73. Kiehl KA, Smith AM, Hare RD, et al. Limbic abnormalities in affective processing by criminal psychopaths as revealed by functional magnetic resonance imaging. Biol Psychiatry 2001;50:677–84.

74. Ledoux J. Synaptic self. New York: Penguin Books; 2003.

75. Lanteaume L, Khalfa S, Régis J, et al. Emotion induction after direct intracerebral stimulations of human amygdala. Cereb Cortex 2007;17:1307–13.

76. Murray EA. Amygdala function in positive reinforcement. The human amygdala. New York: Guilford Press; 2009.

77. Amunts K, Kedo O, Kindler M, et al. Cytoarchitectonic mapping of the human amygdala, hippocampal region and entorhinal cortex: intersubject variability and probability maps. Anat Embryol (Berl) 2005;210:343–52.

78. Bzdok D, Laird AR, Zilles K, et al. An investigation of the structural, connectional and functional sub-specialization in the human amygdala. Hum Brain Mapp 2013;34:3247–66.

79. Aggleton JP, Burton MJ, Passingham RE. Cortical and sub-cortical afferents to the amygdala of the rhesus monkey (*Macaca mulatta*). Brain Res 1980;190:347–68.

80. Brust JC. The practice of neural science: from synapses to symptoms. New York: McGraw Hill; 2000.

81. Groshek F, Kerfoot E, McKenna V, et al. Amygdala central nucleus function is necessary for learning, but not expression, of conditioned auditory orienting. Behav Neurosci 2005;119:202–12.

82. Glascher J, Adolphs R. Processing of the arousal of subliminal and supraliminal emotional stimuli by the human amygdala. J Neurosci 2003;23:10274–82.

83. Phelps EA. Emotion and cognition: insights from studies of the human amygdala. Annu Rev Psychol 2006;57:27–53.

84. Hamann S. Sex Differences in the responses of the human amygdala. Neuroscience 2005;11:288–93.

85. Maren S. Long-term potentiation in the amygdala: a mechanism for emotional learning and memory. Trends Neurosci 1999;22:561–7.

86. Bickart KC, Wright CI, Dautoff RJ, et al. Amygdala volume and social network size in humans. Nat Neurosci 2011;14:163–4.

87. Szalavitz M. How to win friends: have a big amygdala? Time 2010. Available at: http://healthland.time.com/2010/12/28/how-to-win-friends-have-a-big-amygdala/. Accessed April 1, 2016.

88. Qiao Y, Xie B, Du X. Abnormal response to emotional stimuli in male adolescents with violent behavior in China. Eur Child Adolesc Psychiatry 2012;21:193–8.

89. Pardini DA, Raine A, Erickson K, et al. Lower amygdala volume in men is associated with childhood aggression, early psychopathic traits and future violence. Biol Psychiatry 2014;75(1):73–80.

90. Moul C, Killcross S, Dadds MR. A model of differential amygdala activation in psychopathy. Psychol Rev 2012;119(4):789–806.

91. Mufson E, Mesulam MM, Pandya DN. Insular interconnections with the amygdala in the rhesus monkey. Neuroscience 1981;6:1231–48.

92. Yoder KJ, Porges EC, Decety J. Amygdala subnuclei connectivity in response to violence reveals unique influences of individual differences in psychopathic traits in a nonforensic sample. Hum Brain Mapp 2015;36:1417–28.
93. Chakravartyhy V, Joseph D, Bapi R. What do the basal ganglia do? A modeling perspective. Biol Cybern 2010;103(3):237–53.
94. Wenzel JM, Rauscher NA, Cheer JF, et al. A role for phasic dopamine release within the nucleus accumbens in encoding aversion: a review of the neurochemical literature. ACS Chem Neurosci 2015;6:16–26.
95. Yager L, Garcia A, et al. The ins and outs of the striatum: role in drug addiction. Neuroscience 2015;301:529–41.
96. Devinsky O, Morrell MJ, Vogt BA. Contributions of anterior cingulate cortex to behaviour. Brain 1995;118:279–306.
97. Boccardi M, Bocchetta M, Aronen HJ, et al. Atypical nucleus accumbens morphology in psychopathy: another limbic piece in the puzzle. Int J Law Psychiatry 2013;36:157–67.
98. Schultz W. Reward functions of the basal ganglia. J Neural Transm 2016;123: 679–93.
99. Seguin JR. The frontal lobe and aggression. Eur J Dev Psychol 2009;6:100–19.
100. Berridge KC, Kringelbach ML. Pleasure systems in the brain. Neuron 2015;86: 646–66.
101. Olds J, Milner P. Positive reinforcement produced by electrical stimulation of septal area and other regions of rat brain. J Comp Physiol Psychol 1954;47: 419–27.
102. Hoptman MJ. Neuroimaging studies of violence and antisocial behavior. J Psychiatr Pract 2003;9(4):265–78.
103. Hoptman MJ, Volavka J, Czobor P, et al. Aggression and quantitative MRI measures of caudate in patients with chronic schizophrenia or schizoaffective disorder. J Neuropsychiatry Clin Neurosci 2006;18(4):509–15.
104. Barkataki I, Kumari V, Das M, et al. Volumetric structural brain abnormalities in men with schizophrenia or antisocial personality disorder. Behav Brain Res 2006;169(2):239–47.
105. Muneoka K, Igawa M, Kida J. Stroke notes. Cerebrovasc Dis 2008;26:664–5.
106. Kumari V, Gudjonsson GH, Raghuvanshi I, et al. Reduced thalamic volume in men with antisocial personality disorder or schizophrenia and a history of serious violence and childhood abuse. Eur Psychiatry 2013;28:225–34.
107. Cope LM, Ermer E, Gaudet LM, et al. Abnormal brain structure in youth who commit homicide. Neuroimage Clin 2014;4:800–7.
108. Puri BK, Counsell SJ, Saeed N, et al. Regional grey matter volumetric changes in forensic schizophrenia patients: an MRI study comparing the brain structure of patients who have seriously and violently offended with that of patients who have not. BMC Psychiatry 2008;8(Suppl):s6–12.
109. Wahlund K, Kristiansson M. Aggression, psychopathy and brain imaging–review and future recommendations. Int J Law Psychiatry 2009;32:266–71.
110. Gregory S, Ffytche D, Simmons A, et al. The antisocial brain: psychopathy matters. a structural MRI investigation of antisocial male violent offenders. Arch Gen Psychiatry 2012;69(9):962–72.
111. Yankovsky AE, Veilleux M, Dubeau F, et al. Post-ictal rage and aggression: a video EEG study. Epileptic Disord 2005;7(2):143–7.
112. Anderson NE, Kiehl KA. Psychopathy and aggression: when paralimbic dysfunction leads to violence. Curr Top Behav Neurosci 2014;17:369–93.

113. Thompson P, Hayashi K, Simon SL, et al. Structural abnormalities in the brains of human subjects who use methamphetamines. J Neurosci 2004;24:6028–36.
114. Bertsch K, Grothe M, Prehn K, et al. Brain volumes differ between diagnostic groups of violent criminal offenders. Eur Arch Psychiatry Clin Neurosci 2013; 263:593–606.
115. Husted DS, Myers WC, Lui Y. The limited role of neuroimaging in determining criminal liability: an overview and case report. Forensic Sci Int 2008;179:e9–15.
116. Klasen M, Zvyagintsev M, Schwenzer M, et al. Quetiapine modulates functional connectivity in brain aggression networks. Neuroimage 2013;75:20–6.
117. Franzini A, Broggi G, Cordella R, et al. Deep-brain stimulation for aggressive and disruptive behavior. World Neurosurg 2013;80(3–4):SR29.e11-4.
118. Fuji DE, Ahmed I. Psychotic disorder caused by traumatic brain injury. Psychiatr Clin North Am 2015;37:113–24.
119. Leutgeb V, Leitner M, Wabnegger A, et al. Brain abnormalities in high-risk violent offenders and their association with psychopathic traits and criminal recidivism. Neuroscience 2015;308:194–201.
120. Meixner JB Jr. Applications of neuroscience in criminal law: legal and methodological issue. Curr Neurol Neurosci Rep 2015;15(2):513.
121. Pieri E, Levitt M. Risky individuals and the politics of genetic research into aggressiveness and violence. Bioethics 2008;22(9):509–18.

Workplace Violence

Practical Considerations for Mental Health Professionals in Consultation, Assessment, and Management of Risk

Philip Saragoza, MD[a],*, Stephen G. White, PhD[b,c]

KEYWORDS

- Workplace violence • Targeted violence • Threat assessment • Direct threat

KEY POINTS

- Workplace violence risk consultations focus on potential acts of targeted violence perpetrated by individuals with a connection to the workplace, directed toward others in the workplace.
- Distinctions exist between fitness for duty evaluations and violence risk consultations, the latter occurring in dynamic scenarios in which the opinion of risk shifts depending on case developments.
- Effective threat management requires multidisciplinary teamwork, the careful consideration of available interventions, and awareness of the possibility of risk mitigation interventions having unintended consequences.

INTRODUCTION

In the 1980s, a series of shootings by disgruntled US postal workers and other employees focused media attention on acts of violence in the workplace. Over the past 3 decades, researchers have shed light onto the types of violence that occur in the workplace, the characteristics of individuals who engage in workplace violence, and the contextual factors that may escalate or mitigate the risk of violence. These advances and the accumulated experience of threat assessment practitioners have contributed to the development of industry practices designed to prevent workplace violence. Especially among large employers, multidisciplinary threat assessment and management teams receive, triage, investigate, and respond to scenarios of concern.

Disclosure: S.G. White is an author of the WAVR-21.
[a] University of Michigan Medical School, 2395 Oak Valley Drive, Suite 100, Ann Arbor, MI 48103, USA; [b] Work Trauma Services, Inc, San Francisco, CA, USA; [c] Department of Psychiatry, University of California at San Francisco, 3527 Mt. Diablo Boulevard, #123, Lafayette, CA 94549, USA
* Corresponding author.
E-mail address: saragoza@med.umich.edu

Psychiatr Clin N Am 39 (2016) 599–610
http://dx.doi.org/10.1016/j.psc.2016.07.007
0193-953X/16/© 2016 Elsevier Inc. All rights reserved.

psych.theclinics.com

These practices operate in a complex legal context in which the rights of the involved parties must be considered and balanced. In assessing and managing the potential for workplace violence, employers, and others participating in the evaluation process must first determine whether and how to intervene to ensure safety, yet in a manner mindful of the laws and policies intended to protect the employee of concern. In particular, the employer is subject to claims of invasion of privacy, discrimination, and wrongful termination. In this article, we describe the phenomenon of workplace violence, review important elements in the assessment of workplace violence risk, and provide an overview of threat management, including brief commentary on common legal considerations arising in these situations. For the purposes of this article we do not address the issue of "outsider" threats, for example, those posed by a jealous rejected husband or partner of an employee; however, many of the strategic points presented here still apply in those cases.

WHAT IS "WORKPLACE VIOLENCE"?

Naturally, media coverage of incidents of workplace violence focuses on the most egregious and tragic cases: those involving mass murder, often by current or former employees. In reality, homicide represents the extreme end of a continuum of behaviors comprising workplace violence, has been in steady decline since 1993, and accounts for less than 1% of all violent crimes in the workplace.[1] According to the Occupational Health and Safety Administration[2] workplace violence is defined as any act or threat of physical violence, harassment, intimidation, or other disruptive behavior that occurs at the work site, and may cause physical or emotional harm. Short of homicide and physical violence, other workplace violence behaviors include stalking, threats, bullying, and emotional abuse.[3] Specific individuals are not the only targets of workplace violence. Beyond the obvious severe psychological trauma caused by workplace shootings, aggression and threats of violence cause anxiety, fear, and frustration, with resulting damaged morale and productivity.[4] Direct and indirect victims may suffer stress or burnout, physical health problems, and may ultimately leave an organization.[5]

Acts of workplace violence have been categorized in numerous ways. One major typology divides acts of violence according to the relationship between the perpetrator and the organization (**Table 1**).[3] Type 1 acts account for most workplace violence.[6] A key distinction within this framework is that which exists between type 1 acts of workplace violence and all of the others: that is, in type 1 violence, the perpetrator is a stranger to the victims, whereas in types 2, 3, and 4, the perpetrator has a

Table 1
Categories of workplace violence
Type 1 Violent acts by criminals who have no other connection with the workplace, but enter to commit robbery or another crime.
Type 2 Violence directed at employees by customers, clients, patients, students, inmates, or any others for whom an organization provides services.
Type 3 Violence against coworkers, supervisors, or managers by a present or former employee.
Type 4 Violence committed in the workplace by someone who does not work there, but has a personal relationship with an employee (eg, abusive spouse or domestic partner).

From Rugala EA, Isaacs AR, editors. Workplace violence: issues in response. Quantico (VA): Critical Incident Response Group, National Center for the Analysis of Violent Crime, FBI Academy; 2003.

real or perceived connection to the workplace. Although statistical compilations of the motives for workplace violence are not established, analyses of individual cases suggest the psychological reasons for these more "personalized" types of violence. They may be fueled by real or perceived disputes, rejections, grudges, or extreme beliefs rooted in mental illness.[6] In these scenarios, violence is more likely to be intentional, targeting certain individuals or groups. There is also a greater chance that an observable warning sign had likely reached the employer, and/or a "triggering context" was looming.[3]

Violence is more likely to occur in certain workplaces, often in the form of "type 2" acts, as listed in **Table 1**, where it happens in the course of the employee's execution of his or her ordinary duties. Health care workers, law enforcement professionals, security workers, and those involved in the exchange of goods and money (eg, sales clerks, taxi drivers) experience violence more often, due to the inherent nature of their work as well as the characteristics of their clientele. The violence in these instances is more commonly affective, that is, impulsive and unplanned. Workplace violence in the health care industry has received much attention. Hospital-based medical workers were found to have the highest rate of nonfatal assaults over all other sectors of employment.[3] Ironically, surveys and other studies indicate that health care workers tend to underreport acts of workplace violence for several reasons: the perception that violence is merely "part of the job"[7]; the expectation that nothing will be done, or done effectively, about reported problems; and fear of retaliation in instances in which the perpetrator is a superior of the reporting party.[8] Underreporting is just one reason for the unreliability of statistics on workplace violence. Differing definitions of violence and injury and methodological issues further confound interpretation of the data.[9]

Not only does violence occur more often in certain workplaces, but the nature and magnitude of violent acts also differs across workplaces. For example, the emergency room nurse may frequently experience verbal threats and intimidation from inebriated patients or frustrated family members in overcrowded waiting areas. The patient care attendant in a forensic psychiatric hospital may routinely be charged with managing agitated psychotic patients who become physically assaultive. The airline industry must concern itself with the disruptive passenger who may necessitate an emergency landing, an angry, acting-out crew member, or, extremely rare but most dreaded, the suicidal pilot who may endanger a flight full of passengers. These contextual differences call for different measures for prevention and management of violence, ranging from security procedures (eg, metal detectors at the entry points to hospitals) to staff training on deescalation of volatile people to preemployment screening and thoughtful policies triggering fitness for duty assessment. Professionals involved in assessing risk must also account for these contextual differences between workplaces when considering the scope and impact of potential violence.

WORKPLACE VIOLENCE RISK ASSESSMENT

Before describing issues specific to the workplace, certain more general aspects of violence risk assessment deserve mention. First, violence is contextual, meaning that it arises in and is influenced by circumstances. In turn, persons of concern are not either "dangerous" or "not dangerous." The consideration of whether they might engage in violence must account for the interaction between the individual, with all their inherent characteristics (eg, history of violence, poor coping skills, symptoms of mental illness), their circumstances (eg, financial stressors, social isolation), their environment (eg, provocation from others, including people in the workplace), and potential targets.

Viewed in this way, violence risk is dynamic and subject to influence by a number of factors, including interventions designed to help the potential perpetrator with certain personal problems, to control their behavior, or to protect would-be targets.

Another concept to consider when conducting any type of violence risk assessment is the distinction between affective and predatory violence. Affective violence, as referred to previously, is defined by spur-of-the moment aggression and is rooted in the fight-or-flight response. Individuals who are short-tempered and prone to agitation are more likely to engage in affective violence. In contrast, predatory violence refers to premeditated aggression executed in deliberate fashion, without the autonomic and emotional arousal observed in affective violence. Although affective violence is common in workplace settings, and affective and predatory violence are not mutually exclusive in individual cases, much of the research in workplace violence has more recently focused on predatory, targeted violence. The perpetrators of such acts usually have a connection to the workplace, target an individual or group in the organization, or the workplace itself is a symbolic target.

The "pathway to violence" is a framework for illustrating the process of predatory violence.[10] In this model, an individual develops a motive for violence, often a grievance, and reaches a point of rationalization for violence before progressing through preparatory steps culminating in an act of instrumental violence. Violent delusional and paranoid states may contribute in given cases and do not interfere with the perpetrator being organized in his preparation. De Becker[11] formulated the acronym "JACA" to describe that such individuals consider violence Justified, Alternatives to violence to be inadequate or unacceptable, the Consequences for violence to be worthwhile (even including arrest or death,) and they have the Ability and means to carry out violence. Individuals moving along the pathway to violence may display warning behaviors, such as communicating threats to family or friends, settling their affairs, attaining weapons, or withdrawing from usual routines due to immersing themselves in preparations.

Specific to the workplace context, extensive case study has revealed a common triggering phenomenon for violence: narcissistic injury and its conversion to narcissistic rage. Extreme vulnerability to underlying shame, but felt or expressed as a profound sense of injustice or "disrespect," motivates the violence. Psychologically, the act is often one of self-affirmation, a restoration of self-esteem and pride. Perpetrators of workplace violence have often experienced a triggering event of a major setback at work, ranging from unexpectedly being passed over for a promotion to being disciplined or terminated. The scenario of job loss or its potential is quite common in workplace violence consultations, as are ongoing or unsuccessful claims regarding disability, workplace harassment, or wrongful termination.[6] Individuals vulnerable to narcissistic injury are unable to cope with such setbacks in the manner that more commonly resilient employees demonstrate. Coupled with their often inherent problems adapting to disappointment and loss is their inflated perception of their achievement or value in the workplace, as well as their personal identity being excessively defined by their membership in the organization.[6] These factors contribute to the experience of the setback as humiliating, profoundly unfair, unresolvable, intolerable, and demanding action in response.[12] The feeling of impotence experienced with the narcissistic injury is resolved through vengeance, as these individuals achieve a "sense of final control… by going out in a blaze of glory."[12]

Aside from a job setback, threatened or imminent job loss, numerous other workplace-specific factors should be assessed in conducting a workplace violence risk consultation. These include aspects of the organization's culture that can contribute to agitation and grievances, such as excessive work demands; labor disputes and poor relations between labor and management; management with poor communication and overly punitive and/or inconsistent disciplinary methods, including avoidant managing of difficult individuals; and inadequate security and lack of employee counseling.[3] Organizations should not be blamed for the horrible tragedies inflicted by vengeful employees or others, but they must recognize and should address the internal situational factors that enable violence, as well as the lapses in their prevention protocols that hinder safe as well as fair resolutions of threat scenarios.

Although workplace violence risk assessment does not emphasize psychiatric diagnosis, it is obviously critical to ascertain certain aspects of the mental state of the person of concern. The willingness to sacrifice oneself so as to commit violence, and more generally suicidal ideation, are critical risk factors for violence. Some acts of suicide in workplace violence arise out of depression and the desire to escape pain and loss,[6] whereas others reflect the narcissistic drive to restore potency through infamy and revenge. Case reviews of mass murder and workplace murders have demonstrated higher death tolls in those instances in which the perpetrator committed suicide.[13] Felthous and Hempel[14] point out that nearly all perpetrators of workplace homicide are fundamentally self-destructive. Case studies show that those who do not commit suicide (directly or indirectly) most commonly surrender or are captured without concern for escape or denial of culpability.[14]

Suicidality is just one aspect of mental health that should be assessed in violence risk consultation. Depression can contribute to feelings of desperation and hopelessness and can diminish resiliency to cope with stress. Mania or hypomania can manifest with irritability, grandiosity, volatility and erratic behavior, frequent sources of discomfort and concern when occurring in the workplace, and more frequently posing a risk of affective incidents of violence. Substance use can affect mood and cause disinhibited conduct and impaired work performance. It can also lead to the development of covert behaviors designed to conceal substance use that, when discussed or challenged, may trigger defensive, angry reactions from the at-risk employee. Psychosis, particularly paranoid delusions focused on individuals in close contact, such as coworkers, can steer an individual toward violence when the individual mistakenly perceives that he or she is in danger. A broad spectrum of problematic personality traits is also of concern in violence risk assessment. Individuals prone to anger who struggle to accept responsibility, to handle rejection or criticism, or who generally cope poorly with intense emotion are at risk for escalation to violence in response to triggering events. Entitlement, egocentricity, and disregard for others' feelings or needs may translate into justification for vindictive aggression. In assessing risk, it is not just the presence or absence of psychiatric symptoms or traits that is important, but more so their intensity, trajectory, and malleability in response to available interventions; that is, the dynamic (subject to change) rather than static (fixed) aspects of the would-be perpetrator's mental state.

The dynamism of risk and the fact that serious violence in the workplace is a low-base rate phenomenon are 2 reasons that the goal of workplace violence risk assessment is not to predict violence, but instead to identify and prioritize concerning aspects of a given scenario and translate findings into management strategies. Violence risk factors are categorized as either static or dynamic. In conducting workplace violence risk assessments, while certain static pieces of information may be quite important (eg, a history of stalking and domestic violence in a person of concern who is becoming fixated on a coworker), the emphasis is often on dynamic factors, as they are the focus of interventions designed to minimize the risk of violence. This is one reason to characterize the workplace violence risk assessment more as threat assessment, as opposed to traditional "violence risk assessment" (**Table 2**).

Table 2
Some differences between violence risk assessment and threat assessment

	Violence Risk Assessment	Threat Assessment
Urgency/acuity	Low, usually around scheduled events	High, ongoing situations
Person of concern	Often confined	Freely moving among potential victims
Context	Judicial determinations, for example, release from hospital, release onto probation	Unfolding risk scenario, for example, threatening communications and behaviors toward coworker
Available data	Often extensive	Often limited
Purpose	Predicting and/or mitigating risk; management of perpetrator	Mitigating risk; management of potential perpetrator and protection of victim(s)
Methodology	Actuarial and structured professional judgment (SPJ) instruments	SPJ instruments in concert with multidisciplinary input and collaboration

The goals in a workplace violence risk consultation include formulating a narrative for possible scenarios of violence, based on the assessment, integration, and weighing of risk factors, protective factors, and circumstantial factors. This process ultimately leads to hypotheses regarding the following questions about the person of concern:

1. What is a possible explanation for the behaviors causing alarm?
2. Are there identifiable motives or causes for violent action?
3. What would be the nature, severity, and timeline of any violence?
4. Who would be the likely targets?
5. What actions would mitigate risk?
6. What actions might exacerbate risk?

The assessment can be enhanced through the use of structured professional judgment (SPJ) instruments, guided assessment tools that provide a framework for the evaluator to collect data regarding the presence or absence, relevance, and stability of empirically validated risk factors and protective factors. The evaluator integrates this information before applying clinical judgment in arriving at opinions on the level of concern and recommendations for intervention. SPJ instruments increase the consistency and transparency of assessments by ensuring that the same factors are being considered across cases. In the workplace context, SPJs also provide a justifiable basis for employer decision-making regarding termination and other measures that may later be scrutinized in legal proceedings. Today, the use of evidence-based SPJs in violence risk assessment is a well-established practice. There are now a number of SPJs developed for specific populations or contexts, including the workplace. The WAVR-21 (Workplace Assessment of Violence Risk) is an SPJ designed to assess the risk of targeted violence and related behaviors of concern in workplaces and other organizational contexts.[6] Results of a reliability study showed summary interrater reliability correlations for overall presence of risk factors, risk of violence, and seriousness of the violent act in the fair to good range, similar to those of other SPJ instruments. A rating group of only psychologists produced summary rating of violence risk in the excellent range. Some of the individual items had poor reliability, likely due to both clinical and statistical reasons.[15] Predictive validity studies, the true test of an instrument's ability to correctly identify violent individuals before the fact, are the next step in the development of the WAVR-21, and are under way. Such studies are sophisticated and expensive and require large sample sizes owing to the base rate issue: among those individuals who make threats or create concern, only a very few ever commit a workplace homicide.[16]

An important task for the mental health consultant in violence risk assessments is to gather as much information as possible in developing a perspective about the individual's mental state and the trajectory of his or her conduct, including observable behaviors and other collateral data (eg, hostile or paranoid e-mails sent by the person of concern). It is also critical to carefully consider the accuracy of the information and the reliability of sources of information.[17] Informants may intentionally or unintentionally report information that is partially or wholly untrue, for a variety of reasons,[17] and this may distort the view of potential psychiatric issues in the person of concern. Vetting the accuracy of information is especially important when the consultation is *indirect*, meaning that the person of concern is not interviewed. In such consultations, other individuals, including the potential target of violence, may be interviewed in order to gather more complete collateral information about the individual's mental state and behavior and to cross-reference data from other sources. However, when case information suggests that psychiatric symptoms may be significantly influencing the at-risk individual's conduct, direct assessment can provide valuable clarification and lead to effective interventions addressing mental health.

CASE MANAGEMENT

Violence risk assessment and management are inextricably linked. Even in scenarios in which a major goal of risk assessment is to produce a statistically driven prediction of a certain outcome, the utility of that information exists primarily in its implications for management. In more dynamic consultation contexts, such as workplace violence risk assessments, opinions on risk level and management strategies ebb and flow as scenarios unfold and new information arises (eg, the person of concern's responses to limit-setting or mental health treatment). Responding to and managing volatile situations in the workplace are some of the most anxiety-provoking and challenging tasks faced by employers. This is one reason that a common error in case management is to permit situations of concern to percolate and develop for considerable time before any intervention.

Recognition of the importance of timely, consistent, and reliable responses in dealing with disruptive and potentially violent workplace conduct is a major factor that led to the widespread development of workplace violence prevention policies and procedures. Although there is no legal mandate about the composition of such policies and procedures, the Occupational Safety and Health Administration (OSHA) has identified several key elements of effective workplace violence prevention programs. These include the following: management commitment and employee involvement, worksite analysis to identify sources of risk and gauge efficacy of procedures, hazard prevention and control, safety and health training, and recordkeeping and program evaluation.[2] Effective violence risk prevention programs reduce consequences, such as poor work performance, poor workplace morale, and reduced productivity.[18]

Many scenarios of odd, agitated, or disruptive behavior, or even communicated threats, do not actually pose a high level of risk and are effectively handled by individual supervisors, managers, human resources staff, and/or security personnel. However, multidisciplinary, coordinated responses can enhance the assessment of scenarios of concern, particularly when there are indicators of higher risk and more complex considerations for resolution of the situation. Threat assessment and management teams (TMTs) are now fairly commonplace among large companies, and are an emerging standard in institutions of higher education, having been mandated by law in some states.[19] TMTs usually include staff from human resources, security, risk management, legal counsel, workplace health/employee assistance programs, and mental health risk assessment professionals. Their purpose is to identify situations and persons of concern as early as possible, investigate and gather information, assess the situation, and to manage the situation through the selective use of available resources so as to mitigate risk.

Regardless of the personnel involved in investigating and responding to potentially violent situations in the workplace, a range of interventions are available for managing these scenarios, including "doing nothing" but continuing to monitor the situation. Interventions may be categorized along a continuum from confrontational or punitive to nonconfrontational or benevolent.[10] The goal in case management is for interventions to be effective in reducing risk, usually by virtue of timeliness and appropriate focus on the crux of the problem. However, the dynamic nature of risk gives rise to the issue of unintended consequences, or the "intervention dilemma," that is, the recognition that any intervention has the capacity to reduce risk, not affect risk, or even to intensify risk.[20] A rational threat assessment and management approach avoids cookbook responses and decreases vulnerability to the following important errors[6]:

- Not detecting or underestimating potentially high or imminent risk situations
- Overreacting to low or no risk situations, causing unnecessary disruption
- Misappropriating the organization's time and resources in such situations
- Exacerbating a threat scenario with ill-advised responses that increase risk
- Misapplying interventions, for example, treatment or dispute resolution in situations in which they will have little or no impact

A common erroneous response is for the employer to react punitively or with excessively control-focused methods without considering the potential impact of such disciplinary measures. Although it can be tempting and even justified to suspend or terminate an employee who has been engaging in various forms of misconduct or threatening behavior, doing so without considering the potential for these steps to represent triggering events for the at-risk individual can be perilous. Employers should consider conducting a threat assessment before taking significant disciplinary action against an employee raising concern for violence risk. Emergencies exist, but the prudent move is usually to place an employee on a paid leave of absence (so as not to add to his or her distress and implication of blame) while an investigation is undertaken.

When the decision is made to terminate an employee for conduct, suggesting that he or she poses a risk of violence, employers must recognize that risk is not necessarily eliminated. Every effort should be made to handle termination in a manner that preserves the individual's dignity and offers them the maximum opportunity to save face. When appropriate and available, severance packages may be considered, intended to temporarily bridge the individual to his or her next job. These can include sums of money sufficient to last until new income can be secured, or the extension of health care coverage, which might facilitate the person participating in necessary treatment (or avoid forcing the employee to terminate treatment). Regardless of whether such benevolent gestures are made, employers must also consider security measures. There should be consideration of the need for ongoing assessment of the risk posed by the individual and mechanisms to achieve it, ranging from further supportive contact (eg, "check-in" phone calls) to surveillance for communications or approaches to the workplace, to obtaining protective orders. Considering the pros and cons of these options is a routinely complex matter for threat assessment teams, and engaged consultants.

LEGAL ISSUES IN WORKPLACE VIOLENCE

Employers have a duty to maintain a safe workplace, but must fulfill it while minding protections for employees. Failure to do either can lead to costly litigation. There are numerous foundations for employers' responsibility to maintain a safe workplace. OSHA's "General Duty Clause" requires that the workplace be "free from recognized hazards that are causing or are likely to cause death or serious physical harm" to employees.[21] Employers are required by civil rights legislation to protect employees from harassment, including threats and violence, and if employees suffer injuries in the course of employment they are entitled to workers' compensation benefits. Incidents of workplace violence have led to findings of employer negligence in numerous areas, including hiring or retaining dangerous individuals, negligent supervision and training, and negligent recommendation (eg, misrepresenting an employee's violent tendencies to a prospective employer).

With respect to employee rights, there are limits to the type of information employers can request in hiring or investigations. Employers must manage employee misconduct investigations and procedures in accordance with due process, following company policies and collective bargaining agreements.[6] The Americans with Disabilities Act (ADA) protects employees with disabilities (including a variety of psychiatric conditions, such as personality disorders) from discrimination in all aspects of the employment process, including discipline and termination.

ADA issues are often the focus of fitness for duty examinations, common scenarios in which evaluators encounter concerns about workplace violence. The examinee may have been placed on administrative leave after exhibiting signs of possible mental instability and/or engaging in disruptive or threatening conduct. Employers are permitted to insist on a fitness for duty examination if the inquiry is "job-related" and "consistent with business necessity," a standard fulfilled by "a reasonable belief, based on objective evidence, that: (1) an employee's ability to perform essential job functions will be impaired by a medical condition; or (2) an employee will pose a direct threat due to a medical condition."[22] The factors weighed in consideration of direct threat include the following:

- Duration of the risk
- Nature and severity of the potential harm
- Likelihood that the potential harm will occur
- Imminence of the potential harm

In addition, the threat posed by the individual must be one that cannot be eliminated by reasonable accommodation. Although ADA protections may sound onerous for employers, in reality, courts tend to err on the side of caution when there is legitimate information to support the notion of an employee posing a threat in the workplace. First, an employee who threatens coworkers, for example, may not even be deemed to meet the ADA's definition of a "qualified individual" who can perform the "essential functions" of their job, as interacting with others appropriately may be deemed an essential job function. Second, courts have consistently ruled that violations of workplace conduct policies, especially violent behavior, are not protected under the ADA even if they stemmed from the employee's disability. Yet another interpretation of the ADA that has favored employers in cases of concern for workplace violence has been the notion that it may not be reasonable to accommodate a potential threat if it continues to expose other employees to risk of harm.

Three points are essential for evaluators to keep in mind:

1. Employment law counsel must be involved in decisions about the organization's legal obligations in individual cases.
2. Professional experience and clinical judgment will still be essential (but grounded in empirically established risk factors) in defining risk-related terms, such as "direct threat," "duration," and "imminence."
3. The principle of "safety trumps privacy" and other personal rights is primary, but interveners must be able to justify their actions in the interest of safety that may raise legal exposure for the organization. As many attorneys have said to us, "I would rather defend a wrongful termination case than a wrongful death case."

CASE EXAMPLE

The following vignette illustrates the interaction between psychological factors in an individual of concern and workplace factors culminating in risk of violence:

"Bob" has been a maintenance mechanic at a small college for approximately a year and a half. His performance is average and he is subject to procedural mistakes that he denies are his doing. He is regarded as "prickly" and easily frustrated. His boss, Roger, is inconsistent in his supervision, and especially doesn't like dealing with Bob "because you can't talk to the guy." Bob has said openly, "I never trusted any boss. They are all alike." Coworkers can see that Roger is intimidated by Bob and is not dealing with him. When Bob learned that Roger had advocated for his own cousin to get hired at the college, in a completely unrelated department, he became very agitated and began making comments about "favoritism." He mumbled in the work bay about having been fired once because of "unfair treatment by members of the same family who ganged up on me." He started a "log," documenting Roger's "harassment and discrimination" against him.

When coworkers complained about Bob's increasing suspiciousness and unfounded accusations that they were "helping Roger set me up to get fired," the labor relations representative met with him. Bob got very angry in the meeting, accused the representative of colluding with Roger, and demanded someone else conduct an investigation. The representative felt very frightened of Bob and no longer agreed to meet with him. This led to Bob getting a written notice that his "unprofessional conduct will not be tolerated," that he must control his temper, and that any such "outbursts" in the future would lead to "further disciplinary action up to and including discharge." He was referred to the employee assistance program and recommended that he get into an "anger management" program. Bob taped the letter to the door of Roger's office, and wrote on it, "No wonder people come into work and blow everyone away! This is the kind of shit that makes them do it!" He then left the building. As management considered what to do next, Bob called in later and claimed he was suffering "emotional distress and anxiety" from being harassed and was unable to work.

In this case, Bob's perceptions and behaviors at work very likely stem from paranoid issues. Naturally mistrustful and defensive, especially under stress, he is not easy to help or manage with normal supervisory actions. Perceiving malicious intent where none exists leads to further anger on his part and increased avoidance by his boss. His display of problematic behaviors in the workplace for quite some time before any action was taken is a common scenario. Concern is another signal that assessment is warranted.

Somewhat predictably, Bob makes a veiled threat in response to receiving a disciplinary letter, but then claims emotional distress, actually a good sign from a threat assessment view because it implies a deescalation, that he is not in a "nothing to lose" mindset. This suggests several possibilities, including that he is ambivalent about violence, has no real violent intent but was venting or trying to intimidate others, and/or he wants to avoid discipline by declaring himself disabled; his M.O. may be litigious, not violent. In fact, a legitimate claim cannot be ruled out. A violence risk consultant would assist management by assessing any risk posed by Bob, as well as, in this case, evaluating the legitimacy of his stress claim.

Given Bob's susceptibility to shame and subsequent volatility, the entire evaluation response must be handled carefully, and likely include coordinating the assessment process with security measures. Many cases like this one are best resolved by the employee departing the organization, but with a benevolent severance, as mentioned previously, in an attempt to protect his dignity. Returning to the work group is problematic for all parties, as the conflicts cannot be resolved, especially given Bob's nature. The consultant may be helpful to Bob in this regard, noting that a "fresh start" would likely be better for *him*. However, this cannot be done in a manipulative way. The assessor can genuinely empathize with the employee's distress without agreeing with his perceptions, and as an outsider may have some leverage in helping the individual to move on, avoiding a showdown, and perhaps deadly outcome, for everyone involved.

REFERENCES

1. Duhart DT. Violence in the workplace. 1993-99 (NJC 190076). Washington, DC: U.S. Department of Justice, Office of Justice Programs, National Institute of Justice; 2001.
2. United States Department of Labor, Occupational Safety & Health Administration. Workplace violence. Available at: www.osha.gov/SLTC/workplaceviolence/index. html. Accessed May 1, 2016.
3. Rugala EA, Isaacs AR. Workplace violence: issues in response. Quantico (VA): Critical Incident Response Group, National Center for the Analysis of Violent Crime, FBI Academy; 2003.
4. De Puy J, Romain-Glassey N, Gut M, et al. Clinically assessed consequences of workplace physical violence. Int Arch Occup Environ Health 2015;88:213–24.
5. Rogers KA, Kelloway EK. Violence at work: personal and organizational outcomes. J Occup Health Psychol 1997;2(1):63–71.
6. White SG, Meloy JR. The workplace assessment of violence risk (WAVR-21). 2nd edition. San Diego (CA): Specialized Training Services, Inc.; 2010.
7. Stene J, Larson E, Levy M, et al. Workplace violence in the emergency department: giving staff the tools and support to report. Perm J 2015;19(2):113–7. Available at: http://dx.doi.org/10.7812/TPP/14-187. Accessed April 14, 2016.
8. Blando J, Ridenour M, Hartley D, et al. Barriers to effective implementation of programs for the prevention of workplace violence in hospitals. Online J Issues Nurs 2015;20(1):1–16.
9. Schat ACH, Frone MR, Kelloway EK. Prevalence of workplace aggression in the U.S. workforce. In: Kelloway EK, Barling J, Hurrell JJ, editors. Handbook of workplace violence. Thousand Oaks (CA): Sage Publications; 2006. p. 47–89.
10. Calhoun FS, Weston SW. Contemporary threat management: a practical guide for identifying, assessing and managing individuals of violent intent. San Diego (CA): Specialized Training Services, Inc.; 2003.

11. De Becker G. The gift of fear and other survival signals that protect us from violence. New York: Dell Publishing, a Division of Random House, Inc; 1997.
12. Menninger W. Uncontained rage: a psychoanalytic perspective on violence. Bull Menninger Clin 2007;71(2):115–31.
13. Lester D. Murder-suicide in workplace violence. Psychol Rep Disabil Trauma 2014;115(1):28–31.
14. Felthous AR, Hempel A. Combined homicides-suicides: a review. J Forensic Sci 1995;40(5):846–57.
15. Meloy JR, White SG, Hart S. Workplace assessment of targeted violence risk: The development and reliability of the WAVR-21. J Forensic Sci 2013;58(5):1353–8.
16. Hart SD, Logan C. Formulation of violence risk using evidence-based assessments: the structured professional judgment approach. In: Sturmey P, McMurran M, editors. Forensic case formulation. Chichester (United Kingdom): Wiley-Blackwell; 2011.
17. Van Der Meer B, Diekhuis M. Collecting and assessing information for threat assessment. In: Meloy JR, Hoffmann J, editors. International handbook of threat assessment. New York: Oxford University Press; 2014. p. 54–66.
18. Peek-Asa C, Casteel C, Rugala E, et al. Workplace violence investigations and activation of the threat management teams in a multinational corporation. J Occup Environ Med 2013;55(11):1305–11.
19. Nolan J. Addressing intimate partner violence and stalking on campus: going beyond legal compliance to enhance campus safety. Inside the minds: emerging issues in college and university campus security. United States. Thomson Reuters/Aspatore; 2015. p. 4–49.
20. De Becker G. A white paper report: Intervention decisions: the value of flexibility. Paper presented at the annual meeting of the Association of Threat Assessment Professionals. Anaheim, CA. 1994.
21. United States Department of Labor, Occupational Safety & Health Administration. OSHA Act of 1970, SEC. 5. Duties. Available at: https://www.osha.gov/pls/oshaweb/owadisp.show_document?p_table=OSHACT&p_id=3359. Accessed May 1, 2016.
22. US Equal Employment Opportunity Commission. Enforcement guidance:disability-related inquiries and medical examinations of employees under the Americans with Disabilities Act (ADA). Available at: https://www.eeoc.gov/policy/docs/guidance-inquiries.html. Accessed May 1, 2016.

Mental Illness and Firearms
Legal Context and Clinical Approaches

Debra A. Pinals, MD[a],*, Lisa Anacker, MD[b]

KEYWORDS

- Gun violence • Mental illness • Risk assessment • Risk management
- Gun control legislation • Firearms • Media

KEY POINTS

- Despite media stories to the contrary, persons with mental illness account for only a small percentage of persons who commit acts of violence, and an even smaller percentage of persons who commit gun violence toward others, although the risk of individuals with mental illness using firearms for suicide is a significant concern.
- Gun laws and gun registries can provide delays in firearms access and prohibitions to access, but do not eliminate all risk or all access related to firearms, and thus clinicians should be mindful of more individualized risk assessments.
- Sound risk assessment and risk management practices for individual patients in treatment contexts can be helpful in thwarting untoward negative consequences involving suicide or violence.

INTRODUCTION

Tragic events over recent years have heightened awareness and concerns related to gun violence in general, as well as specific concerns related to gun violence perpetrated by persons thought to have mental illness. Separating myth from reality about the risks of gun violence for persons with mental illness becomes especially complicated given numerous recent media reports that continue to emphasize the relationship of mental illness to violence over and above that known in the literature.[1] High-profile, specific incidents of firearm shootings and multiple victims leave the public with an even greater sense that mental illness is a major factor in most mass murder. These representations run a serious risk of increasing stigma against individuals with mental illness who might never commit violence, and without recognition of the potential collateral consequences of this stigma to their lives and the lives of their families. Increasing reports of so-called active shooters have been made in recent years, and across the world it seems the alerts are everywhere.[2]

[a] Program in Psychiatry, Law, and Ethics, Department of Psychiatry, University of Michigan, 4250 Plymouth Road, Ann Arbor, MI 48109, USA; [b] Department of Psychiatry, University of Michigan, 4250 Plymouth Road, Ann Arbor, MI 48109, USA
* Corresponding author.
E-mail address: dpinals@med.umich.edu

Psychiatr Clin N Am 39 (2016) 611–621
http://dx.doi.org/10.1016/j.psc.2016.07.013
0193-953X/16/© 2016 Elsevier Inc. All rights reserved.

For mental health professionals practicing in the United States, it is important to understand the current context related to these media reports, the current legal underpinnings of firearms rights as well as the clinical implications of these rights, and the currently known data related to firearms and mental illness. From there, clinical practice can be informed to best identify those rare cases in which a patient may be at risk of firearm-related violence and cases involving suicide risk with eye toward thoughtful and comprehensive risk assessments. This article offers a review of those areas.

CURRENT CONTEXT WITH REGARD TO MEDIA REPORTS ON FIREARMS AND MENTAL ILLNESS

It is hard to imagine how individuals who are sane can engage in mass murder. Some individuals who have engaged in mass violence might have had some legitimate broad-based mental health issue that makes the extrapolation seem logical. Some might even have had frank mental illness. These individuals, although rare, are the current concerning "needle in the haystack" for clinicians who need to be prepared to conduct proper risk assessments in their clinical practice and work within the parameters of the law related to notifications, firearms access rights, and the like. A few examples that highlight these issues include recent cases that have raised questions about the mental health system and approaches to individuals at risk.

More than 15 years ago, on April 20, 1999, Columbine High School in Colorado made national news when 2 young men, one of whom had been treated for depression, entered carrying firearms and other weapons and fired at students and teachers, killing 13 people with numerous others injured.[3] In 2007, on the Virginia Polytechnic Institute and State University campus, 32 people were killed with many others wounded, after Mr Seung-Hui Cho opened fire, and eventually killed himself.[4] This man had been involuntarily committed to outpatient treatment 2 years before the incident, but the ability to track him and ensure adherence, and the ability to identify him as a person prohibited from acquiring firearms because of that prior commitment, was lost in complex legal and system challenges.[4,5] The presumed protections had proved to have more problems than solutions, and raised numerous questions about how firearm purchases were being monitored and overseen. A complete review of Virginia commitment laws[6] followed and resulted in local statutory commitment reform.[7]

Other noteworthy tragedies included the mass murder of 12 people and concomitant injury of 70 others in a movie theater in Aurora, Colorado, in 2012. James Holmes, the perpetrator in that incident, went through a lengthy trial in which his mental state was at issue, although he was ultimately found guilty.[8] The situation was predated by his having seen a university psychiatrist who, according to reports, had become concerned about his homicidal thoughts and had notified police of concerns, raising questions about the interplay between mental health and law enforcement in potential active threat situations.[9,10]

Later in 2012, the world saw yet another example of mass shooting when Adam Lanza entered an elementary school in a small town called Newtown, Connecticut, after having killed his mother. At the school, he fired shots that killed 20 children and 6 adults before killing himself. In this case, too, the perpetrator's emotional state became a major focus of the public story, and reports indicated that he may have had autism spectrum–type symptoms for which school supports may have been lacking.[11]

These incidents received major media attention, and, as such, it became difficult to balance issues of firearms and safety, especially in the context of mental illness. However, it has been well established that mental illness does not account for most of the violence in society.[12,13] What is not listed in this article are the many stories in which mental illness is not a factor in gun violence. As the debate unfolds regarding risks, many people argue that the best protection for any risk of gun violence is through having greater access to guns for protection. Others seek tighter gun control for all. These debates about gun control have only become more heated over time. To provide an overview of the issues pertaining to mental illness, this article next reviews some of the legal factors related to gun ownership.

LEGAL FACTORS RELATED TO GUN OWNERSHIP, ESPECIALLY RELATED TO MENTAL ILLNESS

The Second Amendment of the United States Constitution reads "A well regulated Militia, being necessary to the security of a free State, the right of the people to keep and bear Arms, shall not be infringed."[14] This Amendment was written in 1791 by founding fathers who had, in the previous decade, seen the end of the Revolutionary War and the establishment of the United States as an independent country. However, even more than 200 years later, the language of this Amendment continues to garner considerable debate.

Before the United States Supreme Court's landmark 2008 decision in *District of Columbia v. Heller*, the court had yet to definitively address this debate.[15] There were, before the *Heller* case, 2 principal opposing theories as to what rights the Amendment protected: the first consisted of an individual rights theory, whereby the Amendment protected an individual's constitutional right to firearm ownership, possession, and transportation. The second theory, often seen as a states' right or collective right concept, argued the Amendment's phrasing of "a well regulated Militia" only protected the right to keep and bear arms in connection with organized state militia units for defense. In the *Heller* case, the plaintiffs challenged the constitutionality of a Washington D.C. handgun ban called the Firearms Control Regulations Act of 1975.[16] The law, with some exceptions, generally banned residents in Washington D.C. from possession of handguns and also required residents to keep any lawfully owned firearms, such as registered long guns, "unloaded and dissembled or bound by a trigger lock or similar device" if in the home.[15] The Court therefore considered whether the prohibition on the possession of usable handguns in the home violated the Second Amendment to the Constitution. They ultimately decided that the phrasing of the Amendment "to keep and bear Arms" could naturally be interpreted to mean "have weapons," and that the Second Amendment protected this right to have weapons as an individual right unconnected with militia service.[15] Supporters of an individual's right to bear arms saw this ruling as a victory for self-defense in the home, individual autonomy, and for personal safety.

Despite the *Heller* decision, as noted earlier, the debate about gun ownership and gun regulation in the United States has not diminished. Debate as well as public concern about those with mental illness purchasing a firearm are not new. Parameters and limitations regarding those who should be prohibited from purchasing a firearm were put in place as early as 1968 with the Federal Gun Control Act.[17] A timeline related to the history of gun control legislation in the United States is delineated in **Fig. 1**. The Federal Gun Control Act, which was passed in the context of the assassination of John F. Kennedy, was intended to regulate interstate transfers of firearms. It created categories of persons prohibited from shipping, transporting, possessing, or receiving a gun, including illegal aliens, those addicted to a controlled substance, noncitizens, and felons. Notably, any person "who has been adjudicated as a mental defective or has been committed to any mental institution" was also prohibited.[17]

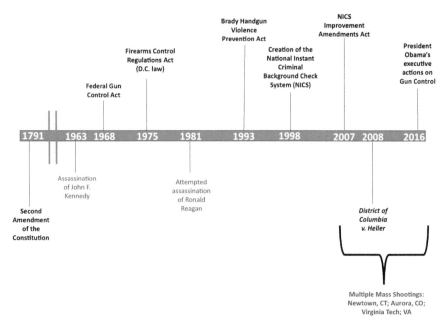

Fig. 1. Timeline of key firearms-related events and legislation in the United States; time not to scale.

This Act required firearms dealers to ask some questions to determine eligibility to purchase firearms.

Following an assassination attempt on President Reagan, which led to the wounding of then White House Press Secretary James Brady, firearm regulation debate returned to the national stage. The Brady Handgun Violence Prevention Act (the so-called Brady Act) was passed in 1993 and, for the first time, established background checks and required a waiting period of 5 days before allowing individuals to purchase a handgun.[18] The Brady Act mandated the creation of the National Instant Criminal Background Check System (NICS) in order to form a national database that would allow background checks and identification of those who were prohibited from purchasing a firearm.[19] The NICS system was launched by the Federal Bureau of Investigation in 1998.[19] As of 1998, when an individual pursues a license to carry a firearm, a review of the NICS database, along with an individual's criminal records, civil restraining orders, and arrests, should occur. Based on this review, an individual is either allowed eventually to obtain the license or is deemed ineligible to make a purchase.

The NICS has led to more than 700,000 denials based on ineligibility criteria since its inception.[19] However, concerns and challenges remain. A major challenge is the lack of consistency regarding state reporting to the national database, because there remains no mandatory requirement to report to NICS. Motivation to report might be greater with federal grant incentives, which were put in place through the NICS Improvement Amendments Act of 2007.[20] This Act was established in the context of the Virginia Tech shooting. As noted earlier, the Virginia Tech shooter was not prohibited from buying a firearm, because there was no information on his prohibiting mental health history in the NICS database.[21]

Although the creation of the NICS database was partially intended to identify and prevent immediate inappropriate firearms purchases, even with a database and more consistent reporting by states there is no guarantee that firearms will not be acquired illegally and used. Obtaining guns from family members or friends bypasses the safety that a database and background checks could provide, and is difficult to control. One study found that 62% of violent gun crime and 28% of gun suicides involved individuals not legally permitted to have a gun.[22]

Specifically with regard to mental health exclusions, the laws apply prohibitions on purchasing a firearm generally to those individuals who have been adjudicated in a court or by an administrative body as having presented as a risk of harming self or others, or being unable to manage their affairs secondary to mental illness.[17] Those who are in mental hospitals or institutions voluntarily or for observation are not included, although states are free to make their own rules regarding reporting requirements. In addition, state practices vary as to the point at which the involuntary status begins within an intervention. For example, there has been debate about whether emergency holds and pick up orders, even if they do not result in commitment, might constitute a trigger for database reporting.[23] There has also been variation between states regarding seizure of firearms. For instance, after conducting an investigation to establish probable cause and determining that no reasonable alternative exists to prevent harm, a Connecticut law allows law enforcement officials to obtain warrants and seize guns from any individual who poses an imminent risk of injuring self or others.[24] However, the law does not specify alternatives or codify specifics about investigations, leaving several areas of implementation of the statute open to interpretation.[24] The idea of gun violence restraining orders has gained some positive attention as a risk management strategy like Connecticut's law, allowing the seizure of a firearm after a court order is issued once the potential for dangerousness is identified. California passed such legislation[25] in the aftermath of another highly publicized mass shooting, in which the family reported few options despite their son's increased risk.[26]

President Obama responded to the highly publicized gun violence by executive action in January of 2016. These actions include, but are not limited to, increasing the number of agents in both the Bureau of Alcohol, Tobacco, Firearms and Explosives (ATF) and the FBI and increasing the efficiency and scope of background checks.[27] Obama also addressed mental illness in his executive actions, calling for increased funding to help those with mental illness receive treatment.[27] He noted that individuals with mental illness are more likely to be the victims of violence than the perpetrators,[27] which is a noteworthy comment that stood in contrast with a public perception of people with mental illness as dangerous.

GUN VIOLENCE TO SELF AND OTHERS AND CLINICAL RISK FACTORS

What is the risk of gun violence by persons with mental illness? Research supports that there is increased risk of injury and death by virtue of increased firearms access alone.[28] Specific to violence and suicide, it is well established that individuals with mental illness who do commit acts of violence with guns are more likely to use that firearm to commit suicide than for interpersonal violence.[29] Firearm-related suicides are a significant clinical concern. Data show that, of suicide deaths, almost half were related to firearms.[30] Therefore, concerns about suicide should be kept at the forefront of examination of risk-reduction interventions related to firearm use.

What about violence directed outward? Studies estimate that general violence toward others attributable solely to people with mental illness makes up only 3% to 5% of violence in the United States.[12,13] Some of the same data examining risk of general violence provide guidance specific to firearm-related violent acts among persons discharged from psychiatric hospitals. A study of the data on the use of firearms

1 year after discharge from acute psychiatric units across multiple sites indicated that only approximately 1% of the patients who had committed violence used guns toward strangers.[31] Of those discharged patients who did use a gun, the individuals also seemed to be cycling through the justice and mental health systems and therefore represented a particular subset of the general population of acutely hospitalized persons.

Attempting to single out mental illness as a major cause of gun violence is therefore misguided, with little supportive evidence. Instead, research has identified several other elements, including substance use, conviction for prior violent offences, and a history of domestic violence, that are better independent risk factors associated with future violence.[13] Suicidal thoughts/behaviors, psychiatric diagnoses, physical illnesses, childhood traumas, family history, and stressful psychosocial features are all factors that increase risk of suicide, or gun violence against self.[32]

However, for both risk of harm to self or others by means of a firearm, when a patient presents, clinicians must be mindful of how to handle the issue of risk related to firearms should that risk arise. In some states, efforts have been made to limit the communication of physicians with patients about firearms access. These so-called gag laws have been delayed in the courts based on appeals.[33] To date, clinicians continue to operate at various levels of knowledge related to these legislative developments and potential constraints. It is therefore important to stay abreast of legal mandates that can arise that might affect how clinicians do a complete risk assessment to include risk factors related to firearm usage. Practicing clinicians should be familiar with their state requirements, allowances, and prohibitions with regard to patients at risk who have access to, or desire to acquire, firearms. **Fig. 2** shows the statutory elements that may be relevant to these circumstances.

CLINICAL RISK ASSESSMENTS WITH A FIREARM-SPECIFIC FOCUS

As with all patients, it is important to conduct a screening and assessment of the patient's risk. Sophisticated and guided risk assessment tools are available and can

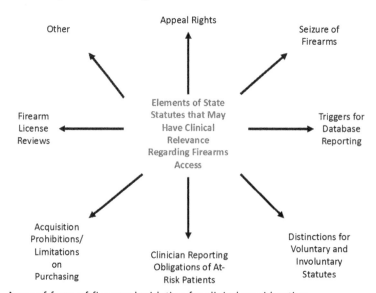

Fig. 2. Areas of focus of firearms legislation for clinical consideration.

be helpful in the right circumstances to help with formalized risk assessments.[34,35] Traditional risk assessments include gathering history and conducting a clinical mental status examination, which are important for baseline information (**Box 1**). Risk factors such as history of violence and assessment of substance use would be encompassed in the generalized history gathering. Although approaches to a full risk assessment are beyond the scope of this article, a review of the history, current ideation, agitation, hopelessness, violent preoccupation, and any collateral sources of information may shed additional light on risk factors and recent activities, patterns of escalation, as well as planned or impulsive violence toward self or others.

For example, one study highlighted the importance of understanding impulsive angry behavior associated with firearm possession as a complex risky combination that might necessitate behavior-based firearms restrictions.[36]

Also, acute and chronic alcohol misuse has been associated with firearm ownership and risk behaviors related to firearms.[37] An assessment of these types of risk factors and current symptoms help provide data to craft a risk-reduction treatment plan. These factors might lead to a conclusion about the level of care needed for these patients during a care episode, what type of monitoring might mitigate risk, and whether care coordination across providers and community support networks needs to be tightened.

As part of a general risk assessment approach with or without a structured guide to professional judgment, clinicians should consider a firearm-specific risk assessment. Practice guidelines from the American Psychiatric Association on general evaluation of adults[38] and on the assessment of suicidal behaviors,[32] as well as other risk management guides,[34,35] are extremely useful clinically, but provide little guidance on what to ask patients with regard to firearms beyond asking about firearm access and safe storage.[32,38] Anecdotal clinical experience in assessing individuals at risk of harm to self and others has shed light on more nuanced approaches that might be taken with regard to patient risk assessment interviews when firearm safety is of clinical concern.

One way of conceptualizing risk assessment related to firearms is to examine what questions are specifically going to yield data that contribute to risk management decisions. After a general risk assessment, a first-tier, or level 1, firearm-specific inquiry might provide more background information that can inform clinical opinion and recommendations. In a level-1 inquiry, a clinician would inquire into basic questions about firearm access, storage, and ammunition availability. An inquiry into the patient's social network can be helpful in guiding whether there are responsible persons who can help in reducing firearm access if needed. A level-2 firearm risk assessment inquiry can be pursued if issues of concern are identified in the earlier questioning. The level-2 questions include an examination of areas of firearm ownership and risk that may be helpful in developing a treatment and risk management plan. **Box 2** delineates specific firearm-focused areas that clinicians may wish to inquire into to help determine the best strategies for risk mitigation over time (see **Box 2**).

Box 1
General clinical risk assessment

- History (biopsychosocial)
- Mental status examination including assessment of risk toward potential targets
- Collateral sources of information

Box 2
Firearm-specific clinical inquiry

Level 1 inquiry

- Firearm ownership
- Firearm access
- Firearm storage
- Ammunition storage
- Social support networks to assist with firearms

Level 2 inquiry

- Acculturation with guns
  - New behavior or interest
- Time spent with gun
- Violent fantasies associated with gun
- Psychodynamic attachment to gun (friends, fears, protection, boredom)
- Hobby/recreational or other intentionality
- Peer/family views

Certain patient groups may have further unique features related to firearms access. For example, for military personnel or law enforcement officers, firearms may become part of the self-identity of the individual, and removal can increase risk more than reviewing firearm safety. Combat exposure was associated with firearms access in one study.[39] This same study suggested that restriction counseling might be helpful for treatment-seeking veterans with combat exposure.[39]

Persons with cognitive disorders may also present complex risks. For example, one study found a high prevalence of firearms in households with family members with dementia and that, in many of those households, guns were kept loaded or family members were unaware of whether the guns were loaded.[40] Youth may also present unique risk factors. For example, high-risk youth who presented in an urban emergency department for assault may have increased rates of subsequent firearm violence necessitating attention to negative attitudes and any behavioral health needs.[41] Gang-related firearm access and culture may also be relevant. Youth may have access with other youth to a hidden so-called community gun and identifying these types of data can be useful in a clinical assessment. Persons with delusional disorders also may harbor ideas about violence that follow the themes of their delusions, and as such inquiries may need to look at concerns through that lens as well. Given the unique angles that each patient presents, practitioners should be comfortable in ascertaining data related to the role of firearms in the day-to-day ideation and life of the patient as part of an overarching risk assessment strategy.

Once risk factors have been identified, treatment planning should make efforts to mitigate such risk. Reporting obligations to public officials and duty to protect third parties are evolving as firearm legislation changes, and, although beyond the scope of this article, a duty of clinicians to take action to protect others (separate from firearm seizure laws) may be mandated by state law.[42] Sherman and colleagues[43] identified the benefits of a comprehensive multidisciplinary inpatient risk-reduction planning process for patients hospitalized with firearm-related suicidal ideation. This planning process included careful assessment as a first step, monitoring that all aspects of the treatment plan have been addressed, providing focused treatment related to dealing with the emotions behind the risk, accessing consultation, and also discharge planning focused on addressing risk factors. The ideas behind this treatment planning process can be generalized to persons who may be at risk of harm to others. Outpatient settings might adopt themes from this comprehensive inpatient approach given that assessment, consultation, and follow-up of risk-reduction efforts makes good clinical sense. Approaches that help clinicians be prepared to deliver counseling about firearms access may also be helpful.[39,44,45] Documentation of risk assessment responses related to firearms access and instructions to patients, suggested in practice guidelines, and documentation of risk-reduction efforts, can be helpful in tracking clinical progress over time and in mitigating liability.[32,38]

SUMMARY

Recognizing that some firearm usage is outside the law, and that the *Heller* decision firmly establishes firearms rights in the United States, efforts toward reduction of morbidity and mortality related to gun violence has shifted to a public health approach.[12] Although most gun violence is not attributable to persons with mental illness, as part of this overall public health strategy, mental health professionals can play a role in reducing gun violence and gun-related suicide on a case-by-case basis through risk assessment, risk management, and awareness of local laws, policies, and practices. These aspects of the general treatment of individuals who may be at risk of suicide or violence are important, even if narrowly focusing public firearms interventions only on individuals with mental illness risks missing a broader population of persons at risk of violence and furthers unreasonable labeling and stigmatization that can thwart efforts to engage persons in need into treatment. General public education, strategic injury and violence prevention, and related research can help guide increasingly effective efforts to reduce gun injury and death on a broader scale over time.

REFERENCES

1. McGinty EE, Kennedy-Hendricks A, Choksy S, et al. Trends in news media coverage of mental illness in the United States: 1995-2014. Health Aff (Millwood) 2016;35(6):1121–9.
2. Pete BJ, Schweit KW. A study of active shooter incidents, 2000-2013. Washington, DC: Texas State University; Federal Bureau of Investigation; US Department of Justice; 2014. Available at: http://www.fbi.gov/news/stories/2014/september/fbi-releases-study-on-active-shooter-incidents/pdfs/a-study-of-active-shooter-incidents-in-the-u.s.-between-2000-and-2013. Accessed November 16, 2014.
3. Columbine High School massacre. Wikipedia. Available at: http://en.wikipedia.org/wiki/Columbine_High_School_massacre. Accessed June 1, 2014.
4. Friedman E. Virginia Tech shooter Seung-Hui Cho's mental health records released. 2009. Available at: http://www.abcnews.go.com/us/seug-hui-chos-mental-health-records released/story?id=8278195. Accessed June 2, 2014.
5. Swartz M, Swanson J. Outpatient commitment: when it improves patient outcomes. Curr Psychiatry Rep 2008;7:25–35.
6. Lo M. Cho's mental illness should have blocked gun sale. 2007. Available at: http://www.nytimes.com/2007/04/20/us/20cnd-guns.html?_r=0. Accessed June 20, 2014.
7. Bonnie RJ, Reinhard JS, Hamilton P, et al. Mental health system transformation after the Virginia Tech tragedy. Health Aff 2009;28:793–804.

8. 2012 Aurora shooting. Wikipedia. Available at: http://en.wikipedia.org/wiki/2012_Aurora_shooting. Accessed July 26, 2014.
9. Connor T. First suit filed against University of Colorado in Aurora shooting. 2013. Available at: http://usnews.nbcnews.com/_news/2013/01/16/16545060-first-suit-filed-against-university-of-colorado-in-aurora-shooting?lite. Accessed June 3, 2014.
10. Morrissey E. Psychiatrist warned campus police about Aurora shooter a month before mass murder. 2013. Available at: http://hotair.com/archives/2013/04/05/psychiatrist-warned-campus-police-about-aurora-shooter-a-month-before-mass-murder/. Accessed June 2, 2014.
11. Griffin A, Kovner J. Adam Lanza's medical records reveal growing anxiety. 2013. Available at: http://www.courant.com/news/connecticut/newtown-sandy-hook-school-shooting/hc-adam-lanza-pediatric-records-20130629,0, 7137229.story. Accessed June 14, 2013.
12. Pinals DA, Appelbaum PS, Bonnie RJ, et al. Resource document on access to firearms by people with mental disorders. Behav Sci Law 2015;33:186–94.
13. Swanson JW. Mental disorder, substance abuse, and community violence: an epidemiological approach. In: Monahan J, Steadman H, editors. Violence and mental disorder: developments in risk assessment. Chicago: University of Chicago Press; 1994. p. 101–36.
14. US Constitution, Second Amendment, 1791.
15. District of Columbia v Heller, 128 S.Ct. 2783, 2788, 2792 (2008).
16. Firearms Control Regulations Act of 1975, D.C. Law 1–85 (1975).
17. Gun Control Act of 1968, 18 USC § 922 (1968).
18. Brady Handgun Violence Prevention Act, Pub L No. 103-159, 107 Stat 1536 (1993).
19. National Instant Criminal Background Check System. The FBI, Federal Bureau of Investigation. Available at: https://www.fbi.gov/about-us/cjis/nics. Accessed July 5, 2016.
20. NICS Improvement Amendment Acts of 2007, Pub L No. 110-180, 121 Stat 2559 (2008).
21. Bureau of Justice Statistics. The NICS Improvement Amendment Acts of 2007, Office of Justice Programs Bureau of Justice Statistics. Available at: http://www.bjs.gov/index.cfm?ty=tp&tid=49. Accessed July 5, 2016.
22. Swanson JW, Easter MM, Roberston AG, et al. Gun violence, mental illness, and laws that prohibit gun possession: evidence from two Florida counties. Health Aff (Millwood) 2016;35(6):1067–75.
23. Hedman LC, Petrila J, Fisher WH, et al. State laws on emergency holds for mental health stabilization. Psychiatr Serv 2016;67(5):529–35.
24. Chapter 529, Division of the State Police. Seizure of firearms of person posing risk of imminent personal injury to self or others. CGS § 29–38c. 2011. Available at: https://www.cga.ct.gov/current/pub/chap_529.htm. Accessed July 14, 2016.
25. California Legislature. Assembly Bill 1014, Chapter 872 Gun Violence Restraining Orders. 2014. Available at: https://leginfo.legislature.ca.gov/faces/billNavClient.xhtml?bill_id=201320140AB1014. Accessed July 17, 2016.
26. Isla Vista Killings 2014. Wikipedia. Available at: https://en.wikipedia.org/wiki/2014_Isla_Vista_killings. Accessed July 17, 2016.
27. The White House, Office of the Press Secretary. Fact sheet: new executive actions to reduce gun violence and make our communities safer. The White House; 2016. Available at: https://www.whitehouse.gov/the-press-office/2016/01/04/fact-sheet-new-executive-actions-reduce-gun-violence-and-make-our. Accessed July 7, 2016.

28. Anglemeyer A, Horvath T, Rutherford G. The accessibility of firearms and risk for suicide and homicide victimization among household members. Ann Intern Med 2014;160(2):101–10.
29. Gold L, Simon R, editors. Gun violence and mental illness. Arlington (VA): American Psychiatric Association; 2016.
30. Murphy SL, Xu J, Kochanek KD. Deaths: final data for 2010. Natl Vital Stat Rep 2013;61:1–117. Available at: http://www.cdc.gov/nchs/deaths.htm. Accessed July 22, 2014.
31. Steadman H, Monahan J, Pinals D, et al. Gun violence and victimization of strangers by persons with a mental illness: data from the MacArthur Violence Risk Assessment Study. Psychiatr Serv 2015;66(11):1238–41. Available at: http://ps.psychiatryonline.org/doi/10.1176/appi.ps.201400512. Accessed July 5, 2016.
32. Jacobs D, Baldessarini R, Conwell Y, et al. Practice guideline for the assessment and treatment of patients with suicidal behaviors. 2010. Available at: http://psychiatryonline.org/pb/assets/raw/sitewide/practice_guidelines/guidelines/suicide.pdf. Accessed July 14, 2016.
33. Lowes R. Florida's 'Gun-Gag' law for doctors upheld by appeals court. Medscape Multispeciality 2014. Available at: http://www.medscape.com/viewarticle/829023. Accessed July 15, 2016.
34. Murrie D. Structured violence risk assessment: implications for preventing gun violence. In: Gold L, Simon R, editors. Gun violence and mental illness. Arlington (VA): American Psychiatric Association Publishing; 2016. p. 221–48.
35. Gold L, Simon R. Decreasing suicide mortality: clinical risk assessment and firearm management. In: Gold L, Simon R, editors. Gun violence and mental illness. Arlington (VA): American Psychiatric Association Publishing; 2016. p. 249–90.
36. Swanson JW, Sampson NA, Petukhova MV, et al. Guns, impulsive angry behavior, and mental disorders: results from the National Comorbidity Survey Replication (NCS-R). Behav Sci Law 2015;33(2–3):199–212.
37. Wintemute GJ. Alcohol misuse, firearm violence perpetration, and public policy in the United States. Prev Med 2015;79:15–21.
38. APA Work Group on Psychiatric Evaluation. The American Psychiatric Association practice guidelines for the psychiatric evaluation of adults. Arlington (VA): American Psychiatric Association; 2016.
39. Smith PN, Currier J, Drescher K. Firearm ownership in veterans entering residential PTSD treatment: associations with suicide ideation, attempts, and combat exposure. Psychiatry Res 2015;229(1–2):220–4.
40. Spangenberg KB, Wagner MT, Hendrix S, et al. Firearm presence in households of patients with Alzheimer's disease and related dementias. J Am Geriatr Soc 1999;47(10):1183–6.
41. Carter PM, Walton MA, Roehler DR, et al. Firearm violence among high-risk emergency department youth after an assault injury. Pediatrics 2015;135:805–15.
42. Soulier MF, Maislen A, Beck JC. Status of the psychiatric duty to protect, circa 2006. J Am Acad Psychiatry Law 2010;38(4):457–73.
43. Sherman M, Burns K, Ignelzi J, et al. Firearms risk management in psychiatric care. Psychiatr Serv 2001;52:1057–61.
44. Johnson RM, Frank EM, Ciocca M, et al. Training mental healthcare providers to reduce at-risk patients' access to lethal means of suicide: evaluation of the CALM Project. Arch Suicide Res 2011;15(3):259–64.
45. Price JH, Kinnison A, Dake JA, et al. Psychiatrists' practices and perceptions regarding anticipatory guidance on firearms. Am J Prev Med 2007;33(5):370–3.

At Risk for Violence in the Military

Stephen N. Xenakis, MD, US Army

KEYWORDS

- Violence • Military • Military culture • Military training • Combat experience

KEY POINTS

- Violence and violent deaths afflict servicemembers, families, and the communities they inhabit.
- Military personnel train for and conduct violent missions to kill the enemy and achieve victory in support of the national interests.
- The military has inherent protective factors and constraints on violence that provide counterbalancing forces.
- Understanding the occurrence and nature of violence in the military entails appreciating military culture, the sociology and demographics of its personnel, military training, combat experiences, and injuries and illnesses that veterans suffer.
- The spillover of violence to the home stations and communities has multiple elements.

INTRODUCTION

Once an army is involved in war, there is a beast in every fighting man, which begins tugging at its chains, and a good officer must learn early on how to keep the beast under control, both in his men and himself.
—General of the Army George C. Marshall – on violence and the Army (1942)

The risk of violence and its tragic consequences for servicemembers and families impinges across the military. Violence and violent deaths afflict servicemembers, families, and the communities they inhabit. Violent behavior and conduct manifests as homicides, suicides, rape, sexual trauma, and spouse and child abuse. Understanding the source and nature of unwanted and illegitimate violence across the military presents unique considerations. The military, as a profession of arms, has distinctive cultural and environmental factors. Military personnel train for and conduct violent missions to kill the enemy and achieve victory in support of the national interests. The American military provides sophisticated training for combat that influences and shapes the psychology of the young warfighter from the moments of first entering active service. The impact and consequences of training and engagement in combat

The Austen Riggs Center, 25 Main Street, Stockbridge, MA 01262, USA
E-mail address: snxenakis@hotmail.com

Psychiatr Clin N Am 39 (2016) 623–631
http://dx.doi.org/10.1016/j.psc.2016.07.008
0193-953X/16/© 2016 Elsevier Inc. All rights reserved.

profoundly influence the attitudes and behavior of servicemembers, raise unique risk factors toward violence, and broadly affect military institutions and the services.

The military has inherent protective factors and constraints on violence that provide counterbalancing forces. Modern warfare follows implicit and explicit rules that guide commanders and warfighters on the ground. Successful military operations, particularly in the twenty-first century, do not involve indiscriminate violence. The doctrine of counterinsurgency institutionalized in Iraq and Afghanistan is based on principles of balance in infantry tactics and building relationships with the local population. As the former commander in Afghanistan, General Stanley McChrystal, stressed, modern warfare requires "courageous restraint" and imposes responsibility on soldiers to know when and where to act.[1] But, war is messy and chaotic, and combat confounds and disorganizes soldiers' attitudes and behavior.

The focus on moral injury highlights the dilemmas facing soldiers on how and where to act violently. Sherman[2] has written on the moral conflicts, psychological state, and attitudes toward violence in the military: "(w)ar is a moral maze about killing and being killed, about liability to lethal and nonlethal harming, about the boundaries of wartime and peacetime, and adapting to the fuzzy boundary crossing."

Understanding the occurrence and nature of violence in the military entails appreciating military culture, the sociology and demographics of its personnel, military training, combat experiences, and injuries and illnesses that veterans suffer. The military is grounded in the principles and practice of conducting violent operations, and the psychology of violence fundamentally anchors its professionalism. The occurrence of unwanted violence and tragic incidence of suicides, homicides, and abuse expose the challenges to containing the behavior outside of the combat and training theaters.

BACKGROUND

In 2009, the Army Medical Department conducted an extensive survey of violent deaths at Fort Carson, Colorado. Eight homicides had allegedly occurred in the previous year perpetrated by 6 soldiers. The Senior Mission Commander, Major General Mark Graham, had initiated a dedicated Task Force in 2008 to investigate the soldiers involved in the incidents and explore the causative factors. The Army and congressional leadership called for a wider review of policies and practices to get to the source of the problems. The Army responded by sending a dedicated team of clinicians and epidemiologists to the Colorado post to conduct an extensive survey and investigation of conditions and environmental factors.

For the preceding several years, the media had focused increasing attention on stories at Army installations on troops returning from the combat theaters. There had been reports of alarming accounts of homicides, suicides, and abuse. A string of murders and suicides had occurred at Fort Bragg and shocked the Army leadership.[2] At least 8 soldiers and family members died by homicide and suicide, and the incidence of serious domestic violence rose sharply. Readers became increasingly aware that soldiers returning from combat in Iraq and Afghanistan were bringing the violence home.[3]

The attention on violent deaths of soldiers heightened with reports of the surprising spike in suicides documented among servicemembers. The Army suicide rate increased dramatically after 2005 while the civilian rate had leveled off. The vast majority of Army suicides were attributed to gunshot wounds. In an attempt to identify risk factors and initiate preventive strategies, the Army allocated $50 million to an extensive Army Study to Assess Risk and Resilience in Servicemembers (Army STARRS).

The potential for violence emerges in families with physical and emotional abuse of children and spouses. The Department of Defense (DoD) has conducted major programs in prevention and treatment of spouse and child abuse for several decades and supported dedicated programs across its installations. Almost all military installations offer Family Advocacy Programs staffed by social workers and other support personnel for the identification, tracking, and treatment of child and spouse abuse.[4] The *Washington Post* reported that DoD confirmed 7676 cases of child abuse or neglect in fiscal year 2014, an increase of 10% from the previous year. Confirmed cases of neglect, which excludes physical and sexual abuse, rose by 14%, military officials said.[5]

More recently, attention has focused on military-related sexual trauma (MRST). The alarming accounts of rapes and sexual assaults has drawn congressional attention and legislative proposals for changes in DoD policies and practices. The overall prevalence of MRST is 7.6% and associated with elevated rates of major depression, posttraumatic stress disorder, and generalized anxiety disorder.[6] Senator Jon Tester (D-Mont.) introduced The Ruth Moore Act in 2015 to ease the processes for veterans who suffered sexual abuse in the military to get help from the Department of Veterans Affairs (VA) and modify the standards for "burden of proof."

EPIDEMIOLOGIC OVERVIEW

The Army has periodically conducted epidemiologic surveys of suicide, violence, and related incidents on installations over the years. The survey of Fort Carson in 2009 stands out as a landmark case. The investigators collected valuable findings on rates and trends of violent deaths and laid the basis for a broader understanding of the nature of violence among military personnel in the garrison environment.[7] The US Army Center for Health Promotion and Preventive Medicine deployed an epidemiological consultation (EPICON) team to investigate common threads among homicide perpetrators, factors unique to Fort Carson, the fraction of waivers among perpetrators, the relationship between deployment and risk factors for violence, and the adequacy and effectiveness of behavioral health services. The EPICON survey represents the most in-depth examination of violent crimes in the Army in the context of community behavioral health risk factors and combat exposure.

The analysis of the cases uncovered findings that have broader implications for understanding untoward events among military personnel:

1. From 2005 to 2008, 13 soldiers at Fort Carson were charged with homicide, attempted homicide, or accessory to homicide.
2. Common threads identified among the index cases included unit of assignment, deployment/combat exposure, military occupational specialty, and behavioral risk factors.
3. Most index cases were assigned to one particular unit.
4. More than 80% of the index cases had deployed at least once to the combat theater. The soldiers deployed had experienced higher levels of combat intensity then other companion units.
5. Half of the cases that deployed and redeployed did not receive normal reintegration training.
6. Half of the index cases were infantry soldiers, and 5 had received enlistment waivers.
7. A high prevalence of behavioral risk factors appeared in the index cases, including substance abuse, diagnoses for mental health conditions, and criminal activity while on active duty.

8. The index cases were at high risk for negative behavioral outcomes, including contributing factors of mental illness, past history of violence and criminal behavior, and substance abuse.
9. Index cases had a higher likelihood of exhibiting misconduct more than other soldiers who deployed in the same units.

The analysis of environmental factors at Fort Carson and the installation revealed important findings and trends:

1. The rates of arrest for major crimes increased across the Army from 2003 to 2009, with the highest rate increase from 2007 to 2008.
2. The arrests for rates increased at Fort Carson from 2006 to 2008.

The epidemiologic team concluded that

1. The soldiers who deployed with the index unit experienced greater combat intensity than comparison units.
2. Those soldiers experienced higher levels of postemployment behavioral health problems, traumatic brain injury, and positive tests for illicit substances.
3. The survey indicated that increasing levels of self-reported combat intensity associated with increased risk for self-reported acts of aggression, problematic alcohol use, criminal conviction, behavioral health problems, and engaging in physical altercations.
4. The focus groups revealed a strong theme of soldiers using alcohol and drugs to "self-medicate."
5. Many soldiers who tested positive for illicit substances did not receive appropriate referrals for evaluation and treatment for substance and alcohol abuse.
6. Soldiers granted waivers for alcohol/drugs or serious nontraffic offenses had a higher likelihood to test positive for listed substances and to be discharged from the Army for misconduct.
7. The survey identified significant barriers to receiving appropriate and timely behavioral health services.

The EPICON concluded that soldiers implicated in criminal activity related to homicide demonstrated risks for engaging in violent behavior based on a cluster of factors, including behavioral health problems, psychopathology, and misconduct. Neuropsychiatric conditions, including alcohol/drug disorders, mood disorder, anxiety disorders, and traumatic brain injury, presented clear risk factors for aggression. Nearly 80% of alleged perpetrators for homicide and related violence had documentation of alcohol or drug abuse, and fewer than half had received appropriate evaluation and treatment. The alleged perpetrators clustered within one particular index unit and had experienced higher levels of combat intensity. The survey indicates an association between increasing levels of combat exposure and risk for negative behavioral outcomes. Although not conclusive, the findings of this Army survey clearly implicated a combination of individual, unit, and environmental factors that converge to increase the population at risk for committing homicide and violence.

SUICIDE

Nearly 2000 soldiers have committed suicide since the first combat engagements in 2001. The words "contagion" and "epidemic" are often used to describe the losses, but the causes and contributing factors have eluded investigation despite the efforts of medical researchers and the Army leadership. The former Vice Chief of Staff of the

Army, General Peter J. Chiarelli, initiated a major review and analysis in 2010 to mitigate the problem. The Army Health Promotion, Risk Reduction, and Suicide Prevention report published under his direction in 2010 documented that more soldiers died as a result of high-risk behavior in the previous year than had died in combat.[8] The report concluded the following:

1. Individuals, families, friends, and leaders have the opportunity to intervene along the care continuum to mitigate suicide and equivocal deaths with an understanding of high-risk behaviors.
2. High-risk behaviors include abuse of alcohol and illicit substances and behavioral health problems.
3. The greatest increase in military suicides has occurred among soldiers who experienced the highest levels of combat intensity.
4. The manner of death determination may underestimate the actual incidents and extent of the problems.
5. The perceived stigma for seeking behavioral health treatment constitutes a real barrier to decreasing the suicide rate. The soldiers most likely needing behavioral health care are the least likely to seek treatment.
6. The relevant risk factors include medical conditions, high-risk behavior, life conditions, and stresses in relationships. The comorbidity of multiple medical conditions, including traumatic brain injury, increase the risk for suicidal behavior.
7. Early recognition and intervention of legal, medical, and disciplinary risk factors present opportunities to prevent negative outcomes. Early detection of behavioral health conditions reflects a willingness to begin treatment and better resolution of symptoms.

The Army STARRS identified multiple factors associated with a high incidence of suicide among military personnel. Nock and colleagues[9] reported that one-third of postenlistment suicide attempts are associated with preenlistment mental disorders. Their studies indicated that reenlistment onset rates among soldiers were lower than civilian cohorts, whereas postenlistment onset of ideation correlated with episodes of intermittent explosive behavior. The documentation of higher fatality rates among Army suicide attempts spotlights the importance controlling the means of suicide, such as availability to and familiarity with firearms. The studies implicate a higher incidence of behavioral health problems and troublesome behavior among soldiers who attempted suicide while on active duty.[10] The incidence of suicide attempts correlates with long-standing observations that mental disorders are leading causes of morbidity among US military personnel.[11]

The extensive and multiple epidemiologic studies sponsored by Army STARRS do not identify specific causative factors for suicide attempts among soldiers.[12] They confirm a steadily rising rate of suicide attempts and deaths from suicide since the beginning of the Iraq and Afghanistan conflicts. The findings constitute potentially useful indicators for preventive strategies but do not help inform clinicians on identifying and intervening with soldiers at risk.

None of the studies comment on the contributing effects of concussions, IED blasts, sleep problems, chronic pain, or co-morbid medical conditions on suicide, mental health problems, and duty performance. The constellation of combat intensity, stress, sleep disruption, injuries, and pain comprise the prevailing experience and reality of servicemembers in combat. The data and findings on concussions, related injuries, and intensity of combat await analysis by the researchers.

CHILD AND SPOUSE ABUSE

Military families experience unique environmental and social factors that influence quality of life and the nature of their relationships.[13] The impact of the Global War on Terror and engagement of military personnel on repeated deployments to Iraq and Afghanistan have uniquely influenced military families and community life.[14] The intensity of combat and repeated deployments to the combat theater have inflicted multiple direct and indirect stresses on the lives of the servicemembers and their families. Psychopathology and the emotional adjustment in military children and families has been linked to the continuous impact on the military at war since 2001.[15] Findings indicate that parental combat deployments impose multiple and cumulative consequences and psychological distress on children. The cumulative length of parental deployments during the child's lifetime correlates with increased risk for depression and externalizing symptoms in the children. A consistent finding of developmental literature has been the association of children's and parental distress, demonstrated again by the findings that 30% to 40% of military parents experience depression and anxiety.

The DoD reported marked increases in the confirmed cases of child abuse in 2014.[5] The DoD data indicate a steady increase in cases from 2008 and contrasts with concurrent declines in rates of abuse in the civilian population. The data require further analysis to identify the characteristics of the families and victims of abuse and neglect reported by the DoD. The DoD has not compiled data on the correlations of numbers and kinds of deployments of servicemembers, prevalence of anxiety, depression, and other emotional disorders with the incidence of child and family abuse, despite the relevant findings over many years.

The presence of psychopathology in abusers of children, spouses, and intimate partners has been documented extensively.[16] Many parents who abuse children and spouses have verified histories of being victims of abuse themselves. Victims of abuse in childhood and adolescence have higher incidence of depression, anxiety, substance abuse, and related disorders. As such, physical abuse constitutes a form of violence that begets violence for subsequent generations.

The causation and antecedents of child and family abuse is multifactorial and complicated. Multiple environmental and social factors contribute to the incidence of child, family, and spouse abuse. Stresses associated with employment, finances, standard of living, and stability in relationships impact the likelihood and nature of abuse. Multiple modalities are used in clinical practice to treat abusers and victims, including the identification and interventions for problems with substance abuse and behavioral health problems that commonly occur.

The Army Health Promotion, Risk Reduction, and Suicide Prevention documented the fragmentation of mental health services across the Army and DoD, including prevention and treatment services for child and family abuse.[8] The gaps in health care services impact formulating and providing coordinated care for servicemembers likely to commit abuse of children and family members and treating contributing conditions, such as alcohol and substance abuse, posttraumatic stress disorder, and postconcussion syndrome. There appears to be an absence of relevant data across the DoD and implementation of integrated programs.

MILITARY SEXUAL TRAUMA

The Congress and news media have spotlighted a rising incidence of sexual assault across the military. Despite the drop in rates across the DoD in recent years, the documentation of nearly 19,000 cases indicates that sexual assaults constitute a significant problem and reflect a disturbing aspect of the military's "organizational culture."[17] The public statements by the DoD do not indicate that the leadership has studied the links between deployments of service members, incidence of psychopathology and other health consequences of combat, and sexual assault in contrast to the VA that has published relevant findings.[17] It is reasonable to assume that the causation of military sexual assault is multifactorial and involves elements of organizational climate, policies for prevention and reporting, and individual contributing factors, including psychopathology and comorbid medical conditions.

SUMMARY

The history of warfare from ancient times recounts vivid tales of returning soldiers, their agony and hardships, and their plunging into violence and despair. More than 14 years of combat in Iraq and Afghanistan involving 2.7 million men and women reaffirms the impact of war on the individual warriors. The violence of war cannot be contained to the battlefield and spills over to the families and communities of the returning soldiers. Violence erupts in many forms when soldiers come home. The rising incidence of suicides among returning servicemembers has become the signature indicator. Additional indicators include highly worrisome reports of homicide, violent crime, risky behavior, accidents, family violence, and sexual assault. The occurrence of such troubling conduct and events is expected among a population of young men and women attracted to the military and volunteering for combat duty. The services rely on the temperament and instincts of the young recruits toward violence to prepare and train the force. Despite the dedicated training that all servicemembers receive on the rules of engagement, containing the occurrence of violence to the special conditions and circumstances of combat comprise a formidable challenge.

A survey of programs and policies across DoD since 2001 uncovers few initiatives to prevent and contain untoward conduct and violence among returning servicemembers. The Army specifically declined to institute decompression programs to facilitate the adjustment of returning soldiers in 2009. Unlike the military services of several European countries and Canada, the United States does not practice formalized decompression and readjustment to assist with the transition from the combat theater. The series of repeated deployments for many soldiers presents serious risks for untoward conduct and violence.

The failure to anticipate the adverse conduct and health consequences of combat on servicemembers ignores the history of warfare and well-recognized lessons learned. In part, the absence of effective policies and practices can be attributed to the current climate across medical and social research. The guidance for military medicine is reductionist and grounded in the predominant principles and thinking on evidence-based approaches across health care research. Accordingly, evidence-based research has translated into conclusions strictly based on empirical findings of narrow studies, but lacks relevance to clinical practice and real-world situations.

The principles of true evidence-based practice involve the integration of best-available research, clinical judgment, and individual preference.[17] These principles apply to understanding the nature and occurrence of violence across the DoD in servicemembers, their families, and their communities. The best-available research goes beyond formal studies and scientific projects and extends to thoughtful reading and understanding of the history of war. Plain and good judgment compels leaders and military medical researchers to acknowledge that many young returning warriors have required dedicated interventions to comprehend the impact of combat duty and reset their personal lives and careers to noncombat environments. The glaring prevalence of drug and alcohol abuse across the range of misconduct related to violence points to the compelling need to design more effective interventions for prevention and treatment. The customary practice across the Army of subjecting young soldiers who use illicit substances to dishonorable discharges from duty merely transfers the problems to the VA and the country at large. Such practices do not protect Americans or heal the damaging consequences of combat.

The spillover of violence to the home stations and communities has multiple elements and appeared tragically during the extended years of these wars. The military, and the nation, are responsible to document the nature and impact of such violence, capture the lessons learned once again for future generations, and act to protect the health and welfare of the citizens who go to war and who live in their communities on returning.

REFERENCES

1. Sherman, N. Making peace with war: healing the moral injuries of war. 2014.
2. Sherman N. AFTERWAR: Healing the Moral Wounds of Our Soldiers. Oxford: Oxford University Press; 2015.
3. Kristof N. When war comes home. The New York Times 2012.
4. DoD Directive 6400.1.
5. Ryan M. The number of child abuse cases in the military hits a decade high. Washington Post 2015.
6. Klingensmisht K, Tsai J, Mota M, et al. Military sexual trauma in US Veterans: Results From the National Health and Resilience in Veterans Study. J Clin Psychiatry 2014;75(10):e1133–9.
7. Epidemiologic Consultation No. 14- HK-0B1U-09, Investigation of Homicides at Fort Carson. Colorado, November 2008–May 2009.
8. U.S. Army. Health promotion, risk reduction, and suicide prevention. 2010.
9. Nock MK, Stein MB, Heeringa SG, et al. Among soldiers: results from the army study to assess risk and resilience in servicemembers (Army STARRS). JAMA Psychiatry 2014;71(5):514–22.
10. Kessler RC, Heeringa SG, Stein MB, et al. Thirty day prevalence of DSM-IV mental disorders among nondeployed soldiers in the US Army: results from the Army Study to Assess Risk and Resilience in Servicemembers (Army STARRS). JAMA Psychiatry 2014;71(5):504–13.
11. Ritchie EC, Benedek D, Malone R, et al. Psychiatry and the military: an update. Psychiatr Clin North Am 2006;29(3):695–707.
12. Schoebaum M, Kessler RC, Gilman SE, et al. Predictors of suicide and accident death in the Army Study to Assess Risk and Resilience in Servicemembers (Army STARRS): results from the Army Study to Assess Risk and Resilience in Servicemembers (Army STARRS). JAMA Psychiatry 2014;71(5):493–503.
13. Jensen PS, Xenakis SN, Wolf P, et al. The military family syndrome revisited: "by the numbers." Presented at the Annual Meeting of the American Academy of Child and Adolescent Psychiatry, October 1988.
14. Carey B. Those with multiple tours of war overseas struggle at home. The New York Times 2016.
15. Lester P, Peterson K, Reeves J, et al. The long war and parental combat deployment: effects on military children and at-home spouses. J Am Acad Child Adolesc Psychiatry 2010;49(4):310–20.

16. Kaplan SJ, Pelcovitz D, Salzinger S, et al. Psychopathology of parents of abused and neglected children and adolescents. J Am Acad Child Psychiatry 1983; 22(3):238–44.
17. Steenkamp MM. True evidence-based care for posttraumatic stress disorder in military personnel and veterans. JAMA Psychiatry 2016;73(5):431.

Understanding Homicide–Suicide

James L. Knoll IV, MD

KEYWORDS

- Homicide • Suicide • Murder • Violence • Psychological autopsy
- Homicide–suicide

KEY POINTS

- Homicide–suicide is the phenomenon in which an individual kills 1 or more people and subsequently commits suicide, usually within a short period of time.
- A subtype of homicide–suicide, mass murder–suicide, is gaining increasing attention, particularly in the United States.
- This article proposes a standard classification scheme that further delineates mass murder–suicides.
- Future research should use the full psychological autopsy approach, to include collateral interviews.

INTRODUCTION

Homicide–suicide (HS) is an act of murder of 1 or several individuals that is followed not long after by the suicide of the perpetrator.[1,2] The subsequent suicide most often occurs within a 24 hour period. Despite its rare occurrence, it has profoundly devastating effects on family and community. The dramatic nature of HS frequently captures media attention, and efforts at recognition and prevention have received much less consideration. The event leaves no living victim or perpetrator, making a clear understanding and subsequent research difficult. Nevertheless, efforts have been made to provide new insights into the phenomenon and to better distinguish it from homicide or suicide alone.[3,4]

The rate of HS varies around the world.[5] In the United States, rates range from 0.134 to 0.55 per 100,000.[2,6–9] HS is responsible for approximately 1000 to 1500 deaths annually in the United States alone.[10] Most research to date suggests that perpetrators of HS differ from the typical murderer or suicide in terms of sociodemographic characteristics.[8] In fact, research findings generally suggest HS has unique characteristics distinguishing it from both homicide only and suicide only, while also

Division of Forensic Psychiatry, SUNY Upstate Medical University, 600 East Genesee Street, Suite 108, Syracuse, NY 13202, USA
E-mail address: knollj@upstate.edu

Psychiatr Clin N Am 39 (2016) 633–647
http://dx.doi.org/10.1016/j.psc.2016.07.009
0193-953X/16/© 2016 Elsevier Inc. All rights reserved.

Abbreviations	
HS	Homicide–suicide
MINI	Mini International Neuropsychiatric Interview
MMS	Mass murder–suicide

sharing certain characteristics with these 2 events.[3] For example, perpetrators of HS are usually older than the average homicide-only perpetrator, and more likely to be married or recently separated.[4] Although perpetrators are most often male, victims are most often female. HS seems to be more likely to be precipitated by interpersonal crises than suicide only.[11] The influence of alcohol and drug abuse seems to be less prevalent in HS as compared with homicide or suicide alone.[4,12]

This article reviews the evidence for establishing a standard classification scheme for HS. In this typology, mass murder–suicide (MMS) is considered a type of HS that is further classified and delineated into a workable subtypology. Because the subject of MMS has been receiving increasing attention, particularly in the United States, its unique psychological and sociocultural aspects are discussed. Finally, preventive methods and future research directions are suggested.

HOMICIDE–SUICIDE CLASSIFICATION

The National Violent Death Reporting System is a US Centers for Disease Control and Prevention database that collects information on all violent deaths and suicides. However, using such a database to study HS has proven problematic owing to the lack of a unique code for HS,[13] which in part stems from an ongoing lack of a universally accepted classification system. In 1992, Marzuk and colleagues[10] proposed a practical and logical clinical typology for the classification of HS. Their system categorizes perpetrators based on victim–perpetrator relationship, and by class of precipitants or motives. For example, virtually all HS research indicates that the most common type of HS is the killing of a woman by her estranged male partner after a breakdown of the relationship.[7,14,15] Marzuk and colleagues classified this type of HS as "amorous jealousy." Depression was the most common diagnosis among these perpetrators, who also had a history of chaotic, abusive relationships with partners.[16] The underlying motivation in this type of HS seems to be the real or threatened loss of a previous intimate partner. This occurs in the setting of "domestic desperation," with the perpetrator likely experiencing feelings of hopelessness and a marginalized identity.[17]

Another type of HS per the Marzuk and colleagues classification is the spousal HS of the "declining health" class. This type involves a man, typically elderly, who kills his spouse and then himself because of deteriorating health of either or both. Beginning in approximately the late 80s and 90s, younger couples suffering from AIDS were also classified in this group. It has been argued that in some cases of the declining health type of HS, the motive may be less of an act of love or mercy, and more of an act of fatalism influenced by depression and desperation.[18] Other types of HS per this classification system (observed with less frequency) are filial, familial, and extrafamilial types. Filicide–suicide may involve a depressed and psychotic mother who kills her child in a so-called "extended suicide."[10,19,20] However, research has delineated 5 other potential motives for filicide, including altruistic ("murder out of love," which may be related to psychosis, depression, or serious childhood illness), acutely psychotic (in which the parent kills the child under the irrational influence of psychosis or mania), fatal maltreatment, unwanted child, and spouse revenge.[19,21] Research has found that the most common parental motives for filicide–suicide were altruistic and acutely psychotic.[20] The spousal revenge motive involves a parent killing a child in a deliberate attempt to make the other spouse suffer.[22] In addition, proof or suspicion of infidelity is a common precipitant for spouse revenge filicide. Spousal revenge filicide may be referred to as the Medea complex in older literature. It is named for the Greek myth about Medea, who kills her children in an act of revenge against her husband.[23]

A familicide–suicide (killing of an entire family) is most often committed by a depressed man who views his act as a delivery of the family from continued hardship.[24,25] In addition, there may be actual or delusional suspicions of infidelity.

The extrafamilial type of HS is sometimes referred to as the "adversarial" type, because the event often involves the killing of a perceived enemy who is unrelated to the perpetrator. Adversarial HS typically consists of disgruntled employees, or chronically angry "injustice collectors." These individuals are likely to be suspicious, relatively isolated, and experiencing a recent life crisis. They have a persecutory worldview and seek revenge in the workplace or indiscriminately.[17,25] Mass murderers who commit suicide fit into this category, because their relationships to their victims are often extrafamilial and adversarial in nature.

The reliability of the basic principle underlying the classification scheme from Marzuk and colleagues can be seen in its global consistency. The predominance of the amorous jealousy type, and less frequent occurrence of filicide–suicides and familicide–suicides have been observed regularly over time, as well as internationally.[15,26] The classification scheme suggested in this article includes elements of both the Marzuk and colleagues[10] typology, as well as the approach of Felthous and colleagues.[1] It involves a 2-part label in which the first descriptor denotes the perpetrator's relationship to the victim(s), and the second descriptor specifies causation or motive. The relationship–motive classification scheme has the advantage of conveying maximum information with brevity. A second advantage is flexibility. Research has shown that when HS cases are thoroughly analyzed, they do not always fit cleanly into existing classification schemes. When HS cases are investigated using the full psychological autopsy method, to include conducting collateral interviews, a more accurate determination of motive can be achieved.[27] The actual motive for a HS may be quite different from the apparent motive suggested by media reports or record review only. Because new events are encountered that do not fit existing categories, new categories may be generated following the formula of relationship–motive. The classification system proposed here is a further extension of the relationship–motive scheme, with modifications based on recent research, as well as updated terminology. For example, the older typology of "amorous jealousy/consortial–possessive" is replaced with intimate–possessive. This updated and proposed typology is outlined in **Box 1**.

THE PSYCHOLOGICAL AUTOPSY AND HOMICIDE–SUICIDE

Previous studies of HS have relied on data gathered from police and coroner's reports.[14,28–30] Although still providing useful data, such studies do not capture important clarifying details such as the nature of precipitating stressors and the presence or absence of psychiatric symptoms demonstrated by the perpetrator. Important variables such as family history of suicide or homicide, psychiatric history, violence history, and other personal risk factors are often missed when only police or coroner's reports are used in research. To date, only 2 studies have used interviews of family members in addition to record reviews to enhance the psychological autopsy approach.[16,27] By using the full psychological autopsy method, the data from HS cases become more complete, making conclusions more accurate.

> **Box 1**
> **Homicide–suicide classification system**
>
> *Classification*
>
> - Relationship + motive
> - Relationship between victim and perpetrator (spousal, familial, etc)
> - Motivation of perpetrator (jealousy, altruism, revenge, etc)
>
> *Major patterns*
>
> I. Intimate–possessive
>   Most common type, accounting for 50% to 75% of all homicide-suicides. Involves a male in his 30s or 40s, recently estranged from his partner. Relationship often characterized by domestic abuse and multiple separations and reunions.
>
> II. Intimate–physically ailing
>   The perpetrator is usually an elderly man with poor health, an ailing spouse, or both. The failing health has typically resulted in financial difficulties. Depression is frequent, and the motive may involve altruism or despair about the future. Suicide notes are often left and describe an inability to cope with poor health, finances, and loneliness.
>
> III. Filicide–suicide
>   About 40% to 60% of fathers and 16% to 29% of mothers commit suicide immediately after murdering their children. Infants, however, are more likely to be killed by the mother. A mother killing a neonate is unlikely to suicide. There are further subtypes of filicide–suicide based on motives, such as psychosis, altruism, and revenge.
>
> IV. Familicide–suicide
>   Involves the depressed senior man of a household. There are often associated precipitating stressors of marital problems, finances, or work-related problems. He may view his action as an altruistic "delivery" of his family from continued hardships. He may also suspect marital infidelity and be misusing substances. There is usually evidence of depression or depressive cognitions distorting judgment. In some rare cases, the perpetrator may begin with familicide and then go on to commit mass murder–suicide.
>
> V. Extrafamilial homicide–suicide
>   Typically involves a disgruntled ex-employee, a bullied student, or resentful, paranoid loner. He externalizes blame onto others, and feels wronged in some way. He is very likely to have depression, as well as paranoid and/or narcissistic traits. Actual persecutory delusions may sometimes be seen. Other variants of this type include disgruntled litigants, patients, or clients. This perpetrator often uses a powerful arsenal of weapons, and has no escape planned. The event may involve a "suicide by cop" in that he forces police to kill him, or otherwise kills himself before police can apprehend him. Many cases of mass murder–suicide fall into this type and can be further delineated using the scheme in **Box 2**.

The psychological autopsy was developed initially to assist coroners in determining cause of death.[31,32] The approach has been used to understand suicides more fully for approximately one-half of a century, and helps to guide public health policy.[33] Psychological autopsies are superior to mere record review because they are more comprehensive and more likely to capture psychological and contextual circumstances preceding the HS.[34] Data are synthesized from multiple sources, resulting in an in-depth understanding of personality, behavior, and motives. Unique and critical individual information may not be present in police or coroner records, which do not typically focus on such data. An example of the importance of conducting collateral interviews to complete the full psychological autopsy was seen in a study of 18 HS cases.[27] A standardized psychological autopsy protocol was used, in addition to a modified MINI (Mini International Neuropsychiatric Interview) to inquire about psychiatric

---

Box 2
Mass murder classification descriptions

Classification scheme

- Relationship/linkage + motive
- Relationship or link between victims and perpetrator (work, school, family, specific community, pseudocommunity, etc)
- Motive of perpetrator (resentful, psychotic, depressed, etc)

Pattern examples

- Workplace–resentful
  Disgruntled ex-employee, or resentful employee who is upset with a supervisor, coworker(s), or some aspect of the work environment. He externalizes blame onto others, and feels wronged in some way. He is very likely to have depression, as well as paranoid and/or narcissistic traits. Actual persecutory delusions may sometimes be seen.

- School–resentful
  Bullied, disaffected, or socially alienated student who is motivated by feelings of rejection or humiliation by peers. Depression and/or suicidal threats are likely to be present before the offense, and the perpetrator often communicates his intent to third-party peers.

- Specific community–resentful
  Includes disgruntled clients or others harboring deep resentment toward an identifiable group, culture or political movement.

- Pseudocommunity–psychotic
  Includes individuals experiencing paranoid or persecutory delusions flowing from a psychotic disorder. They target a group that they delusionally believe is persecuting them. Paranoid psychoses and/or strong paranoid cognitions are common.

- Familial–depressed
  See *familicide–suicide* type in **Box 1**. This type may be used when family victims total 4 or greater. If there is evidence of a psychotic depression, the event may be more properly classified as *familial–psychotic*.

- Indiscriminate–resentful
  Generally rageful, depressed and often paranoid individual who releases his anger arbitrarily in some public place. The victim group may be chosen randomly, or on the basis of convenience or ease of access to large numbers of victims.

---

symptoms observed in the perpetrators. Police reports and narratives were reviewed, in addition to interviewing relatives or close friends of the deceased perpetrator. Although demographic findings were consistent with past research, important factors were identified solely through collateral interviews. These factors included the perpetrators: preoffense threats to commit HS (50%), past violence (78%), family history of suicide (22%), and past psychiatric treatment (22%). Collateral interview was critical in obtaining this data, because it was known only by family or friends and not included in police or coroner reports.

Equally important was the finding that, when HS cases are analyzed thoroughly and collateral interviews are conducted, they do not always fit cleanly into existing classification schemes. For example, 1 case in the above mentioned study involved a grandmother who suffered from both schizophrenia and depression. She had no known history of violence or substance use. Paranoia and depression motivated her to plan to "altruistically" kill herself, her child, and her 3 grandchildren. She barricaded herself, her adult child, and the grandchildren in a garage, which she then set on fire. This case had unique features that would lead to difficulty when attempting to classify it using preexisting systems. Using the classification scheme proposed here, this case would be classified as familial–psychotic. Another case that could not be classified using preexisting systems involved a man who suddenly shot his best friend and then immediately shot himself. It was determined through collateral interview that, at the time of the HS, the perpetrator was experiencing a methamphetamine-induced psychosis that resulted in severe paranoia and delusional beliefs that his friend was persecuting him. Using the classification scheme proposed here, this case would be classified as extrafamilial (friend)–psychotic (substance induced). This case would have remained unclassifiable without the family interview portion of the psychological autopsy technique. Such results highlight the importance of conducting collateral interviews to complete the full psychological autopsy. A fuller appreciation of motive and critical factors that might be relevant to future prevention cannot be achieved without collateral interviews. It is argued that this approach should be used in future research to ensure a more accurate and complete understanding of HS, and particularly MMS.

MASS MURDER–SUICIDE

Mass murder has been defined as the killing of 4 or more victims in a single episode.[35] In a majority of cases, the offense ends with the suicide of the perpetrator.[36] Like HS, mass murder is a rare phenomenon.[37] A 2014 study from the Federal Bureau of Investigation found an average of 11.4 incidents of mass shooting occurred annually, resulting in an extremely low base rate for study.[36] The vast majority of incidents occurred in either a place of business or an educational environment. Perpetrators were overwhelmingly men. A US Secret Service study focusing on school shootings from 1974 to 2000 found that perpetrators had frequently considered or attempted suicide, had easy access to family-owned firearms, and "leaked" their intent to commit the offense to peers in some manner.[38] In addition, they were found to have engaged in behavior before the incident that was, retrospectively, cause for concern (eg, weapon seeking, disturbing writings).

Certain factors are commonly observed among individuals who commit mass murder. These factors include extreme feelings of anger and revenge, the lack of an accomplice (when the perpetrator is an adult), feelings of social alienation, and planning out the offense well in advance.[39] MMS is made more difficult to study because, like HS, the perpetrator cannot be evaluated after the event. In a unique case series study involving detailed forensic psychiatric evaluations of 5 mass murderers who survived by chance, a number of common traits and historical factors were found.[40] The subjects had all been bullied or isolated during childhood, and subsequently became socially isolative and despairing. They demonstrated paranoid traits such as suspiciousness and grudge holding. Their worldview suggested a paranoid mindset, because they believed others to be generally rejecting and uncaring. As a result, they spent a great deal of time feeling resentful and ruminating on past humiliations, which ultimately evolved into fantasies of violent revenge.

Paranoid cognitions can be found frequently in the analysis of individual cases of MMS.[41] However, these paranoid cognitions may or may not rise to the level of psychosis. It is important to keep in mind that there has been no systematic psychological autopsy study of a large sample size of MMS cases. Thus, no clear relationship between psychiatric diagnosis and mass murder has been established.[35] The paranoid mindset discussed here involves 2 important nuances: (1) an association with violence, and (2) dimensionality. Dimensionality refers to the concept that personality traits "can be located on the spectrum of trait dimensions," and so may be present "in different degrees rather than being present versus absent."[42] Thus, paranoia can exist on a continuum. In the case of mass murderers, it may range from chronic suspiciousness to frank psychosis with paranoid delusions.

Like HS, MMS has eluded a broadly accepted classification system. The literature contains descriptors such as family annihilator, school shooter, pseudocommando, and disgruntled employee, among others. These descriptors and their vague boundaries may run the risk of impeding future research. The association of mass murder with suicide of the perpetrator has led to the event being described as "suicide with hostile intent."[43] Thus, in this proposed classification system, MMS is considered a subtype of HS, falling into either the familicide–suicide or the extrafamilial–suicide types. **Box 2** gives a proposed classification system for MMS that is a further delineation of the HS classification scheme outlined in **Box 1**. For MMS classification, the term *linkage* is added to the *relationship* descriptor to emphasize the fact that some perpetrators may have no meaningful interpersonal relationship with their victims, but may have only a connection via some mutually shared activity such as work or school.

The relationship/linkage–motive classification scheme allows for multiple permutations to best describe an individual case. For example, the school–resentful type of mass murderer would include offenders who target schoolmates and have the motive of hostile revenge. Examples of incidents that fit this description include the Columbine and Sandy Hook offenders. The workplace–resentful type describes the aggrieved or disgruntled employee or ex-employee who is upset with a supervisor, coworker(s), or some aspect of the work environment and commits murder in the workplace and then dies by suicide. These individuals typically externalize blame for their problem onto others, and feel they have been wronged. They are very likely to have depression, as well as paranoid and/or narcissistic traits. The indiscriminate–resentful type describes the generally rageful, depressed, and often paranoid individual who vents his or her anger arbitrarily in some public place. The victim group may be chosen randomly or on the basis of ease of access to large numbers of people. An example of this category is the man who shot and killed 22 and injured 19 others at a San Diego McDonalds in 1984.[44] This angry but nonpsychotic man told his wife immediately before the offense that "society had their chance," and that he was leaving to go "hunting humans." No evidence indicated that he felt particularly aggrieved by that specific McDonalds or its employees. Rather, the evidence indicated that he had chosen the location due to his familiarity with it and his knowledge that large numbers of potential victims were likely to be present.

In a seminal paper on mass, serial, and sensational homicides, Dietz[25] described a type of mass murderer he termed the "pseudocommando," who plans out the offense ritualistically and comes prepared with a powerful arsenal of weapons. The proposed MMS classification system describes two types of "pseudocommando" style mass murderers as suggested by Dietz: a specific community–resentful type and a pseudocommunity–psychotic type. Both include individuals who have paranoid character traits and are driven by strong feelings of anger and resentment. The specific community–resentful type describes disgruntled clients or others harboring deep resentment toward an identifiable group, culture or political movement. In contrast, the pseudocommunity–psychotic type involves those experiencing paranoid or persecutory delusions flowing from a psychotic disorder. The essential difference between the two is the presence of paranoid psychosis in the pseudocommunity–psychotic type who delusionally believes a group is systematically persecuting him.

NEW DIRECTIONS IN HOMICIDE–SUICIDE RESEARCH
Late Life Homicide–Suicide

It has been observed that, after a domestic homicide, the older offender frequently commits suicide.[45] Late life HS would most often be classified as the intimate–physically ailing type per the classification scheme in **Box 1**. However, not all older perpetrators fall neatly into this category. The characteristics of older spousal HS may have similarities and differences according to context and culture.[5] Although most data on HS involve those belonging to the intimate–possessive type, there remain limited data on HS committed in late life. In a study of 4 cases of HS in which the perpetrators' ages ranged from 65 to 82 years, all 4 perpetrators were men.[46] Two of the cases could be classified as belonging to the intimate–possessive type, 1 case was of the filicide–suicide type, and 1 case would be classified as fratricide–suicide. All 4 cases were associated with major social crises as precipitants and only 1 case occurred in the context of a psychotic mental illness. Such findings underscore the importance of analyzing age-related biopsychosocial issues in suicide and HS research.

Military Homicide–Suicide

Concern about suicide risk in the military has increased over the past the decade. However, questions about relative risk and specific risk factors remain. For example, deployment may not be associated with increased rates of suicide, whereas separation and dishonorable discharge seem to be associated with an increased risk.[47] Just as there seem to be certain important differences for military suicide risk, it is possible that military HS may differ from civilian HS in certain key ways. In a study comparing 259 military HS with 259 civilian HS, the military perpetrators were found to be older and less likely to abuse substances than civilian perpetrators.[48] Military HS perpetrators were also more likely to have physical health problems and be currently or formerly married. Given military personnel's access to firearms and other special concerns, future research on military HS is needed.

Aircraft Homicide–Suicide

In 2015, the copilot of Germanwings Flight 9525 purposely flew the jetliner into a mountainside, killing himself and 149 other people. Before this incident, plane-assisted suicide was known to occur, albeit rarely.[49,50] The Germanwings 9525 incident drew significant attention to the fact that there was relatively little research on the subject of aircraft-assisted HS. A review of available literature on the subject found evidence for the applicability of HS research to the plane-assisted suicide phenomenon.[51] The vast majority of aircraft HS involves a middle-aged male perpetrator. The authors suggested that social stressors may play a role, in particular divorce, separation, and threats to identity.

A systematic review of 18 cases of aircraft HS involving 732 deaths found that pilots had perpetrated 13 of the HS events.[52] Relative to nonaviation samples, a significant percentage (17%) of pilot suicides were classified as aircraft HS. Five of 6 HS events by pilots of commercial airliners occurred after they were left alone in the cockpit, as was the case in the Germanwings incident. Although no single factor was associated with the risk for suicide or HS, factors associated with both events included legal and financial crises, occupational conflict, mental illness, and relationship stressors.

PREVENTION

There is often doubt about researching and enacting preventive measures for public health concerns that have a very low base rate. Yet this fact alone should not obscure the reality that many potential preventive methods for HS are similar in nature to those already being used for suicide and homicide alone. By studying all facets of HS, as well as its component parts (suicide and homicide alone) the underlying factors contributing to HS and MMS may be better understood.[5] Future research efforts should include the full psychological autopsy method on larger sample sizes. This is necessary to better understand how different subtypes of HS have different commonalities, and thus different implications for prevention.

To better guide research in this area, a widely accepted classification scheme must be used. Through a better understanding of risk factors, prevention may be enhanced in clinical practice. It seems likely that, when subtypes of HS have been more thoroughly understood, different risk factors may emerge for different subtypes. For example, the intimate–possessive subtype seems to have significant overlap with certain domestic violence scenarios. Given the relative high prevalence of male perpetrators and female victims in the setting of an estranged intimate relationship, it has been suggested that future HS research focus on issues of domestic violence and men's mental health.[17] Late life HS and military HS seem to have their own respective key risk factors. Research should also focus on trauma, resilience, and healing among survivors, family, and community where HS and MMS have occurred.

Screening efforts and clinical practice will be enhanced by the understanding of more targeted risk factors that can then be used to implement risk management plans. A better evidence base for specific HS risk factors would also help clinicians to know when to probe for HS ideations in an individual who is initially referred for evaluation of suicidal or homicidal ideation only. The standard suicide risk assessment procedure could then be better tailored to include questions specific to HS. Examples of HS specific risk factors deserving of further research include interpersonal and domestic crises, recent separation, and criminal justice problems.[11,17,53]

Empirical and anecdotal evidence has suggested that practical interventions include (1) third-party reporting of warning behaviors or leaked intent, and (2) social and media responsibility.[54,55] News media coverage after a HS or MMS may use terms such a "mentally ill," "insane," or "deranged" to describe the shooter, often before gathering any definitive information. A study of newspaper reporting of HS found that perpetrators were described in inaccurate and unhelpful ways, with significant speculation about their alleged mental illness.[56] Authors noted that accurate news reporting is essential for reducing the stigma of mental illness, which may in turn encourage people to seek help if they are experiencing similar emotional distress. Significant research data have already shown that erroneous and negative attitudes toward persons with mental illness are widespread in society.[57] Media coverage after collective traumas has been observed to have public health effects, particularly in terms of stress-related symptoms.[58] With increased reliance on social media as a news source, media errors may easily intensify public stress, as well as exacerbate the problem of sensationalizing tragedies.[59]

Perhaps more concerning is the finding of a "contagion effect" after MMS, whereby mass shootings are incented by similar events reported in the media.[60] The increased risk of contagion effect for mass shootings was found to last approximately 2 weeks. It is theorized that the greater the relative media sensationalism, the greater the risk of contagion. This seems to be consistent with the finding that perpetrators often study and idolize past MMS perpetrators who had received sensational news coverage.[40] Thus, interventions designed to improve media responsibility should dissuade this and similar dialogue in the aftermath of a HS or MMS. Efforts to develop a universal reporting code that would appropriately cover the tragedy and reduce the impact of the "copycat" effect have been recommended, and generally include avoiding emphasis on perpetrators. In particular, care should be taken to neither glorify nor demonize them.[61] Indeed, media should avoid much emphasis at all on the perpetrator, while instead emphasizing victim and community recovery efforts. Future research should focus on which elements of media coverage are problematic and which are effective in promoting public health goals.[62]

The issue of gun control is discussed frequently in terms of suicide prevention and mass shootings. This issue is complex and contentious, and a full exploration is beyond the scope of this article. In sum, research has suggested that the United States and nations with similarly high firearm ownership rates are predisposed to mass shootings.[63] Much media and political attention has been given to enacting laws focusing on mental illness and firearm laws in the wake of highly publicized mass shootings. Because the percentage of violent acts that are attributable to serious mental illness is very low[64] (and most of these acts do not involve guns), the contribution to public safety of laws directed toward individuals with mental illness in preventing gun violence is likely to be very small.[65] Few of the current state laws enacted to reduce firearm mortality are actually associated with reduced firearm mortality.[66] This is likely due to the fact that such laws focus on irrelevant or ineffective measures. Instead, policy and law must focus on behaviors associated with increased risk for committing gun violence, as opposed to broad categories such as mental illness or psychiatric diagnoses.[67]

The majority of investigation, particularly involving MMS, has focused on issues of gun control and psychiatric diagnosis. In contrast, there has been comparatively little examination of sociocultural factors.[68] Sociocultural factors may provide critical data for prevention efforts that extend beyond low yield individual factors such as mental illness or efforts to "profile" offenders. For example, there are differences between urban and suburban school shootings, and some acts are likely related to the perpetrator's perception of threats to his social identity.[69,70] Suburban and rural shootings may be characterized by social alienation, whereas urban incidents are typically associated with interpersonal violence. Social marginalization and familial dysfunction are also observed in mass shootings.[71]

The investigation of social and cultural factors seems reasonable, if not obvious, when attention is paid to the words perpetrators leave behind. For example, one mass shooter from Montreal in 2006 wrote: "It's society's fault... Society disgusts me."[72] The Sandy Hook Elementary School shooter posted online in late 2011: "[You know what I hate]... Culture. I've been pissed out of my mind all night thinking about it."[73] The Isla Vista California shooter posted a manuscript online in 2014 stating: "Humanity is a cruel and brutal species."[74] Mullen[40] (2004) keenly observed that perpetrators of mass shootings acknowledged being influenced by previous mass murderers who received significant media exposure. This led Mullen to suggest that a Western cultural "script" may be an important factor contributing to the propagation of these tragic events. Extensive and sensationalistic media attention beginning in the 1990s may have propagated the western "script" described by Mullen, resulting in a perverse glamorization of the act, particularly in the eyes of subsequent perpetrators. The study of individual cases of mass shootings that have occurred since the 1990s suggest that perpetrators often felt socially rejected, and perceived society as continually denouncing them as unnecessary, ineffectual, and pathetic.[39,41] Instead of bearing the burden of perceived humiliation, they plan a surprise attack to prove their hidden "value."

By becoming a lone protestor against an "unjust" reality, the perpetrator creates and assumes a powerful victim role in which he can "win"—even by losing. Western society in particular has had a long-standing fascination with the tragic antihero or the outlaw, for example, the Bonnie and Clydes and John Dillingers of American history.[75,76] Their short, violent lives have become the stuff of romanticized, tragic legend. The very public and dramatic nature of mass murder seems to speak to a "need for recognition from an audience."[77] The staged and exposed act of tragic revenge has the function of establishing a connection with spectators who will not soon forget what they have seen. Thus, a further extension of Mullen's western cultural script may be characterized as the *script of the tragic antihero*, which consists of the following "acts":

1. The perception of a ruined social identity;
2. The experience of persecution and social alienation;
3. The formulation of plans to reclaim the identity via tragic revenge;
4. The need for the tragic revenge to be dramatic/theatrical in nature;
5. The public enactment of tragic revenge; and
6. The aftermath of media coverage and propagation.

The final written communication of the Isla Vista California shooter seems to follow this script precisely. His communications reflect a pattern of alienation and malignant envy, culminating in a violent bid for fame and validation: "Humanity has rejected me…. Exacting my retribution is my way of proving my true worth to the world."[74] Future research into the sociocultural factors associated with HS and MMS will likely suggest more detailed preventive efforts, but the present findings suggest that concerted and early efforts at improving the mental health of children and adolescents would be helpful. For many decades, sexual health education has been taught to teens and adolescents. However, a similar focus and stress on mental health education is rarely seen in children's early education. Well-informed and compassionate education on mental health and mental wellness may not only reduce future stigma, but also serve as a beneficial public health intervention. Such education could become increasingly sophisticated as children progress through school. In particular, this may serve as an early preventive effort, while encouraging more open discussion in schools about important mental health issues.

SUMMARY

HS is a rare and catastrophic event. For researchers and clinicians to achieve a better understanding of HS, it is necessary to obtain collateral information from those who witnessed the perpetrator's behavior before the event. In addition, the full psychological autopsy method should be used to enhance the accuracy of findings. MMS can be considered a subtype of HS, with further classification using the relationship/linkage–motive scheme. For progress to occur, especially in translating research into prevention efforts, a standardized classification scheme should be widely accepted. This article has proposed a foundational system of classification that is both practical and flexible. Future research efforts should focus on the specific subtypes of HS so that clinicians may have a better understanding of when to ask patients about thoughts of HS instead of suicidal or homicidal thoughts alone. Preventive efforts should also focus on social and media responsibility. In particular, media reporting and sociocultural factors must be handled thoughtfully in the case of MMS.

REFERENCES

1. Felthous A, Hempel A. Combined homicide-suicides: a review. J Forensic Sci 1995;40:846–57.

2. Bossarte R, Simon T, Barker L. Characteristics of homicide followed by suicide incidents in multiple states, 2003-04. Inj Prev 2006;12(Suppl II):ii330–8.
3. McPhedran S, Eriksson L, Mazerolle P, et al. Characteristics of homicide-suicide in Australia: a comparison with homicide-only and suicide-only cases. J Interpers Violence 2015. [Epub ahead of print].
4. Panczak R, Geissbühler M, Zwahlen M, et al. Homicide-suicides compared to homicides and suicides: systematic review and meta-analysis. Forensic Sci Int 2013;233(1–3):28–36.
5. Bell C, McBride D. Commentary: Homicide-suicide in older adults–cultural and contextual perspectives. J Am Acad Psychiatry Law 2010;38(3):312–7.
6. Coid J. The epidemiology of abnormal homicide and murder followed by suicide. Psychol Med 1983;13(4):855–60.
7. Milroy CM. The epidemiology of homicide-suicide (dyadic death). Forensic Sci Int 1995;71(2):117–22.
8. Bridges F, Lester D. Homicide-suicide in the United States, 1968-1975. Forensic Sci Int 2011;206(1–3):185–9.
9. Large M, Smith G, Nielssen O. The epidemiology of homicide followed by suicide: a systematic and quantitative review. Suicide Life Threat Behav 2009;39:294–306.
10. Marzuk PM, Tardiff K, Hirsch CS. The epidemiology of murder-suicide. JAMA 1992;267(23):3179–83.
11. Kalesan B, Mobily M, Vasan S, et al. The role of interpersonal conflict as a determinant of firearm-related homicide-suicides at different ages. J Interpers Violence 2016. [Epub ahead of print].
12. Carretta C, Burgess A, Welner M. Gaps in crisis mental health: suicide and homicide-suicide. Arch Psychiatr Nurs 2015;29(5):339–45.
13. McNally M, Patton C, Fremouw W. Mining for murder-suicide: an approach to identifying cases of murder-suicide in the national violent death reporting system restricted access database. J Forensic Sci 2015;61(1):245–8.
14. Malphurs JE, Cohen D. A newspaper surveillance study of homicide-suicide in the United States. Am J Forensic Med Pathol 2002;23(2):142–8.
15. De Koning E, Piette M. A retrospective study of murder-suicide at the Forensic Institute of Ghent University, Belgium: 1935-2010. Med Sci Law 2014;54(2):88–98.
16. Rosenbaum M. The role of depression in couples involved in murder-suicide and homicide. Am J Psychiatry 1990;147(8):1036–9.
17. Oliffe J, Han C, Drummond M, et al. Men, masculinities, and murder-suicide. Am J Mens Health 2015;9(6):473–85.
18. Cohen D, Llorente M, Eisdorfer C. Homicide-suicide in older persons. Am J Psychiatry 1998;155(3):390–6.
19. Resnick PJ. Child murder by parents: a psychiatric review of filicide. Am J Psychiatry 1969;126(3):325–34.
20. Friedman SH, Hrouda DR, Holden CE, et al. Filicide-suicide: common factors in parents who kill their children and themselves. J Am Acad Psychiatry Law 2005;33(4):496–504.
21. Friedman SH, Resnick PJ. Child murder by mothers: patterns and prevention. World Psychiatry 2007;6(3):137–41.
22. Wilczynski A. Child homicide. Oxford: Oxford University Press; 1997.
23. McGraw-Hill Concise Dictionary of Modern Medicine. S.v. "Medea complex." 2016. Available at: http://medical-dictionary.thefreedictionary.com/Medea+complex. Accessed July 31, 2016.
24. Selkin J. Rescue fantasies in homicide-suicide. Suicide Life Threat Behav 1976; 6(2):79–85.

25. Dietz PE. Mass, serial and sensational homicides. Bull N Y Acad Med 1986;62(5): 477–91.
26. Shiferaw K, Burkhardt S, Lardi C, et al. A half century retrospective study of homicide-suicide in Geneva–Switzerland: 1956-2005. J Forensic Leg Med 2010;17(2):62–6.
27. Knoll J, Hatters-Friedman S. The homicide – suicide phenomenon: findings of psychological autopsies. J Forensic Sci 2015;60(5):1253–7.
28. Felthous AR, Hempel AG, Heredia A, et al. Combined homicide-suicide in Galveston County. J Forensic Sci 2001;46(3):586–92.
29. Morton E, Runyan CW, Moracco KE, et al. Partner homicide-suicide involving female homicide victims: a population-based study in North Carolina, 1988-1992. Violence Vict 1998;13(2):91–106.
30. Moskowitz A, Simpson AIF, McKenna B, et al. The role of mental illness in homicide-suicide in New Zealand, 1991-2000. J Forensic Psychiatry Psychol 2006;17(3):417–30.
31. Knoll JLIV. The psychological autopsy, part I: applications and methods. J Psychiatr Pract 2008;14(6):393–7.
32. Scott CL, Swartz E, Warburton K. The psychological autopsy: solving the mysteries of death. Psychiatr Clin North Am 2006;29(3):805–22.
33. Botello T, Noguchi T, Sathyavagiswaran L, et al. Evolution of the psychological autopsy: fifty years of experience at the Los Angeles County Chief Medical Examiner-Coroner's Office. J Forensic Sci 2013;58(4):924–6.
34. Conner KR, Beautrais AL, Brent DA, et al. The next generation of psychological autopsy studies. Part I. Interview content. Suicide Life Threat Behav 2011; 41(6):594–613.
35. Fox JA, DeLateur MJ. Mass shootings in America: moving beyond Newtown. Homicide Studies 2014;18(1):125–45.
36. Blair J, Schweit K. A study of active shooter incidents, 2000–2013. Washington, DC: Texas State University and Federal Bureau of Investigation; U.S. Department of Justice; 2014.
37. Investigative Assistance for Violent Crimes Act of 2012, 28 USC 530C(b)(1)(M)(i).
38. Vossekuil B, Fein R, Reddy M, et al. The final report and findings of the safe school initiative: implications for the prevention of school attacks in the United States. Washington, DC: U.S. Department of Education; Office of Elementary and Secondary Education; Safe and Drug-Free Schools Program and U.S. Secret Service; National Threat Assessment Center; 2002.
39. Knoll J. Mass murder: causes, classification, and prevention. Psychiatr Clin North Am 2012;35:757–80.
40. Mullen P. The Autogenic (Self-Generated) Massacre. Behav Sci Law 2004;22: 311–23.
41. Knoll J, Meloy R. Mass Murder & the Violent Paranoid Spectrum. Psychiatr Ann 2014;44(5):236–43.
42. American Psychiatric Association. Diagnostic & statistical manual of mental disorders. 5th edition. Washington, DC: American Psychiatric Association; 2013.
43. Preti A. School shooting as a culturally enforced way of expressing suicidal hostile intentions. J Am Acad Psychiatry Law 2008;36(4):544–50.
44. Mitchell R. Dancing at Armageddon: survivalism and chaos in modern times. Chicago: University of Chicago Press; 2002.
45. Bourget D, Gagné P, Whitehurst L. Domestic homicide and homicide-suicide: the older offender. J Am Acad Psychiatry Law 2010;38:305–11.

46. Cheung G, Hatters Friedman S, Sundram F. Late-life homicide-suicide: a national case series in New Zealand. Psychogeriatrics 2016;16(1):76–81.
47. Reger M, Smolenski DJ, Skopp NA, et al. Risk of Suicide Among US Military Service Members Following Operation Enduring Freedom or Operation Iraqi Freedom Deployment and Separation From the US Military. JAMA Psychiatry 2015;72(6):561–9.
48. Patton C, McNally M, Fremouw W. Military Versus Civilian Murder-Suicide. J Interpers Violence 2015. [Epub ahead of print].
49. Sinha S. A history of cashes caused by pilots' intentional acts. The New York Times 2015. Available at: http://www.nytimes.com/interactive/2015/03/26/world/history-plane-crashes-pilots.html?_r=0. Accessed May 29, 2016.
50. Aviation Safety Network. List of aircraft accidents caused by pilot suicide. Available at: http://news.aviation-safety.net/2013/12/22/list-of-aircraft-accidents-caused-by-pilot-suicide/. Accessed May 29, 2016.
51. Rice T, Sher L. Preventing plane-assisted suicides through the lessons of research on homicide and suicide-homicide. Acta Neuropsychiatr 2015;28:1–4.
52. Kenedi C, Friedman SH, Watson D, et al. Suicide and murder-suicide involving aircraft. Aerosp Med Hum Perform 2016;87(4):388–96.
53. Holland K, Brown S, Hall J, et al. Circumstances preceding homicide-suicides involving child victims: a qualitative analysis. J Interpers Violence 2015 [Epub ahead of print].
54. Meloy R, O'Toole M. The concept of leakage in threat assessment. Behav Sci Law 2011;29(4):513–27.
55. O'Toole M. A different perspective on the UCSB mass murder. Violence Gend 2014;1(2):49–50.
56. Flynn S, Gask L, Shaw J. Newspaper reporting of homicide-suicide and mental illness. Bjpsych Bull 2015;39(6):268–72.
57. Bizer G, Hart J, Jekogian A. Belief in a just world and social dominance orientation: evidence for a mediational pathway predicting negative attitudes and discrimination against individuals with mental illness. Pers Individ Dif 2012;52:428–32.
58. Holman E, Garfin D, Silver R. Media's role in broadcasting acute stress following the Boston Marathon bombings. Proc Natl Acad Sci U S A 2014;111(1):93–8.
59. Berkowitz D, Liu Z. Media errors and the 'nutty professor': riding the journalistic boundaries of the sandy hook shootings. Journalism 2016;17:155–72.
60. Towers S, Gomez-Lievano A, Khan M, et al. Contagion in mass killings and school shootings. PLoS One 2015;10(7):e0117259.
61. Etzerdorfer E, Sonneck G. Preventing suicide by influencing the mass media reporting: the Viennese experience, 1980-1996. Arch Suicide Res 1998;4:67–74.
62. Schildkraut J, Muschert G. Media salience and the framing of mass murder in schools: a comparison of the Columbine and Sandy Hook Massacres. Homicide Studies 2014;18(1):23–43.
63. Lankford A. Public mass shooters and firearms: a cross-national study of 171 countries. Violence Vict 2016;31(2):187–99.
64. Fazel S, Grann M. The population impact of severe mental illness on violent crime. Am J Psychiatry 2006;163:1397–403.
65. Appelbaum P, Swanson J. Law & psychiatry: gun laws and mental illness: how sensible are the current restrictions? Psychiatr Serv 2010;61(7):652–4.
66. Kalesan B, Mobily M, Keiser O, et al. Firearm legislation and firearm mortality in the USA: a cross-sectional, state-level study. Lancet 2016;387(10030):1847–55.

67. Knoll J, Annas D. Mass murder and mental illness. In: Gold L, Simon R, editors. Gun violence and mental illness. Arlington (VA): American Psychiatric Publishing; 2016. p. 81–104.

68. Flanner D, Modzeleski W, Kretschmar J. Violence and school shootings. Curr Psychiatry Rep 2012;15(1):331.

69. Flannery DJ, Singer MI, Wester K. Violence exposure, psychological trauma, and suicide risk in a community sample of dangerously violent adolescents. J Am Acad Child Adolesc Psychiatry 2001;40:435–42.

70. Brown RP, Osterman L, Barnes CD. School violence and the culture of honor. Psychol Sci 2009;20:1400–5.

71. Newman KS, Fox C, Harding D, et al. Rampage: the social roots of school shootings. 1st edition. New York: Basic Books; 2008.

72. Langan A. I am angel of death, warned college killer. Daily Telegraph 2006. Available at: http://www.telegraph.co.uk/news/worldnews/1528946/I-am-Angel-of-Death-warned-college-killer.html. Accessed January 8, 2015.

73. World Press. Adam Lanza posted about "depression" on the day his mother bought him a gun. 2014. Available at: http://sandyhooklighthouse.wordpress.com/2014/01/18/adam-lanza-posted-about-depression-on-the-day-his-mother-bought-him-a-gun/. Accessed January 8, 2015.

74. Rodger E: My twisted world. 2014 Available at: http://www.documentcloud.org/documents/1173808-elliot-rodger-manifesto.html. Accessed May 30, 2016.

75. Spillane J. Myth, Memory, and the American outlaw. Oral Hist Rev 1999;26(1):113–7.

76. Kunhardt P, Kunhardt P III. Violence: an American tradition. 1995. Available at: http://www.ncjrs.gov/App/publications/abstract.aspx?ID=164419. Accessed July 31, 2016.

77. Neuman Y. On revenge. Psychoanal Cult Soc 2012;17(1):1–5.

The Clinical Threat Assessment of the Lone-Actor Terrorist

J. Reid Meloy, PhD[a],*, Jacqueline Genzman, BA[b]

KEYWORDS

- Terrorism • Risk assessment • Mass murder • Lone actor

KEY POINTS

- The TRAP-18 (Terrorist Radicalization Assessment Protocol) is a structured professional judgment instrument for the assessment of individuals who present a concern for lone-actor terrorism.
- It consists of eight proximal warning behaviors and 10 distal characteristics.
- Previous research has demonstrated its interrater reliability and some concurrent and postdictive validity.
- TRAP-18 is retrospectively applied to the case of a US Army psychiatrist and jihadist, Malik Nidal Hasan, who committed a mass murder at Fort Hood, Texas, in November 2009.
- The strengths and limitations of TRAP-18 as a structured professional judgment instrument for mental health clinicians are discussed, and clinical risk management suggestions are made.

Although there are many definitions of terrorism, and ideologies that drive such acts of violence toward noncombatant civilians, they share two common characteristics. First, they are acts of targeted violence, intended and purposeful events that are virtually always the culmination of a pathway toward violence. Acts of terrorism are not impulsive, and typically not a reaction to an imminent threat, which define most violence among individuals.[1,2] Second, not only is a target selected, but an audience, as noted by Bakunin, the nineteenth century anarchist, in his definition of terrorism as "propaganda of the deed." Recent attacks by jihadists against Westernized democracies, most notably in Paris, San Bernardino, Nice, Orlando and Brussels, have underscored the degree to which the audience is anyone who has access to television, the Internet, or social media.

[a] San Diego Psychoanalytic Center and Department of Psychiatry, University of California, San Diego, La Jolla, CA, USA; [b] Department of Psychology, University of Nebraska-Lincoln, Lincoln, NE, USA
* Corresponding author.
E-mail address: reidmeloy@gmail.com

Psychiatr Clin N Am 39 (2016) 649–662
http://dx.doi.org/10.1016/j.psc.2016.07.004
0193-953X/16/© 2016 Elsevier Inc. All rights reserved.

One of the counterterrorism responses has been to search for a means by which lone-actor terrorists can be identified in real time before they act by efficiently organizing accumulating data. Such approaches have encountered several problems: (1) the traditional finding in violence risk research that historical variables are the best predictors has less relevance to lone-actor terrorists[3]; (2) the lack of efforts to draw a distinction between affective (emotional, reactive, impulsive) violence and predatory (instrumental, intended) violence,[4] the latter mode of violence being the domain of terrorists; (3) the lack of attention to proximal and dynamic factors as the best predictors of short-term violence risk, and distinguishing them from more long term, distal characteristics, although this seems to be changing; and (4) the conflation of prediction and prevention. From an epidemiologic perspective, prevention does not require individual prediction, as long as risk factors are known. The paradox is that if prevention is effective, whether primary or secondary, one will never know which individuals would have become symptomatic (or in this application, carried out an act of terrorism) if no intervention had been done.

We believe the young scientific discipline of threat assessment and threat management can alleviate some of these issues,[5] and has a direct application to mental health professionals in their clinical work. First developed by the US Secret Service 20 years ago,[6,7] threat assessment focuses on behavioral facts that may be dynamically changing in real time to determine which individuals pose a risk of targeted violence. It is distinctive in many ways from traditional violence risk assessment, which is a more static approach to determine general violence risk.[8] Since its inception, threat assessment has been successfully used in several risk domains, including stalking, public figure approaches and attacks, workplace violence, school violence, university violence, and adolescent and adult mass murder.[5] The threat assessment model is being used by local, state, and federal law enforcement agencies in various countries to address the risk of targeted violence, including terrorism.

One practical method may eventually provide a reasonable assessment of risk of individual terrorism, based on the recommended domains of Monahan[3,9] and incorporating work on proximal warning behaviors for targeted violence[10-12]: the Terrorist Radicalization Assessment Protocol (TRAP-18), an investigative template developed for operational purposes. This article explores the use of TRAP-18 as a structured professional judgment instrument for clinical use by mental health professionals.

TRAP-18 consists of two sets of variables: first, eight warning behaviors that were originally developed to identify patterns of proximal risk for intended or targeted violence, in contrast to the more common mode of violence, which is typically impulsive or reactive.[1,13] Second, 10 distal characteristics of the lone-actor terrorist were derived from studying the extant empirical and theoretic research on terrorism and Meloy's experience as a forensic psychologist[10,14] in directly and indirectly assessing foreign and domestic lone-actor terrorists over the past 20 years.[15] The proximal warning behaviors and distal characteristics are listed in **Box 1**.

There are two distinctive aspects to TRAP-18, however, which are worth noting. First, TRAP focuses on patterns of behaviors, rather than discrete variables. We think this is a more productive clinical approach that guards against a myopic, and perhaps misleading focus on one risk variable. Second, the two components of TRAP (proximal warning behaviors and distal characteristics) allow the mental health professional to make a determination as to whether the case should be actively managed (the presence of one or more warning behaviors) or just continue to be monitored (a cluster of only distal characteristics). This distinction utilizes the work of Monahan and Steadman[16] who drew from the weather forecasting research concerning

---

Box 1
TRAP-18 (Terrorist Radicalization Assessment Protocol) indicators

Proximal Warning Behaviors

Pathway

Fixation

Identification

Novel aggression

Energy burst

Leakage

Direct threat

Last resort

Distal Characteristics

Personal grievance and moral outrage

Framed by an ideology

Failure to affiliate with an extremist group

Dependence on the virtual community

Thwarting of occupational goals

Failure of sexual-pair bonding

Changes in thinking and emotion

History of mental disorder

Creativity and innovation

History of criminal violence

Watching and Warning and applied this distinction to violence risk assessment. Although there is a strong theoretic underpinning for TRAP-18,[12,15] ongoing empirical testing is needed to demonstrate its reliability and validity. The current status of such studies is as follows:

- Criterion validity of the warning behaviors: This has been demonstrated in several samples of targeted violence cases, including nonterrorist attackers of German public figures,[17,18] spousal homicide perpetrators, US Presidential and political attackers and assassins, school attackers and school threateners,[19] European individual terrorists,[20] and individual case studies.[21,22]
- Postdictive validity of the warning behaviors: This has only been demonstrated in one study,[23] wherein a comparison of school shooters and other students of concern found significant differences with large effect sizes between the two samples for pathway, fixation, identification, novel aggression, and last resort. The students of concern who ultimately had no intent to act violently had virtually none of these five warning behaviors.
- Criterion validity of TRAP-18: This has been demonstrated in two studies, a sample of 22 European individual terrorists,[20] and a sample of 111 European and North American lone-actor terrorists.[24] There is one interrater reliability study[25] for TRAP that indicates an overall mean kappa coefficient of 0.895, with a range of 0.691 to 1.0.

- Generalizability of TRAP-18: This has been demonstrated in Meloy and Gill[24] in the equivalence across most indicators when comparing samples of jihadists, right wing extremists, and single issue terrorists. There was also equivalence with the exception of one indicator (previous violent criminal behavior) when comparing lone-actor terrorists and autonomous cells in Europe.[20]
- Postdictive validity of TRAP: There is some support for this in the identification of four indicators on the instrument that discriminated between thwarted and successful lone-actor terrorists; effect sizes were small to medium.[24]

We demonstrate the clinical usefulness of TRAP-18 as a structured professional judgment instrument by applying it to the case of Nidal Malik Hasan, a US Army psychiatrist and jihadist who committed a mass murder at Fort Hood, Texas, in November 2009. We define each indicator of TRAP-18, followed by the behaviors of Dr Hasan, which illustrate the indicator. Although serious clinical and operational mistakes were made in this case, we acknowledge that we are now privy to evidence in the public domain that was not available to those involved in the case at the time; and it is easy, because of the ubiquity of hindsight bias, to believe that such an act was clearly predictable, when it was not. Given the extremely low base rate for ideologically motivated killing (there have been about 150 murders by all terrorists in the United States since 9/11[26] in contrast to 22 handgun murders *per day* in the United States because of other motivations) such events are not predictable, but we think they are preventable.

CASE SYNOPSIS

Nidal Malik Hasan was born in Virginia on September 8, 1970. His parents had emigrated from Palestine, and he grew up in a moderate Muslim household. Hasan enlisted in the US Army after high school, despite his parents' misgivings. In 1997, he entered the Uniformed Services Medical School; Hasan's parents died young and in short succession during his first few years of medical school.[27] The 9/11 terrorist attacks occurred 2 years before Hasan earned his medical degree. Hasan then went on to complete his psychiatric residency at Walter Reed Army Medical Center, along with a Masters of Public Health and a fellowship at the Uniformed Services University of Health Sciences, the military's chief medical institution; both sites are located near the nation's capital in Bethesda, Maryland. After receiving a promotion to Major in May 2009, Hasan was transferred to Fort Hood in Texas. He arrived in July 2009 with the understanding that deployment was imminent. The official notification came in October for a November deployment to Afghanistan.[28]

Hasan, age 39, attacked the Fort Hood Readiness Processing Center on November 5, 2009, the day his unit was to report there for predeployment medical evaluations. He left his apartment at 6:00 AM to attend morning services at a local mosque before returning to his apartment and giving away several belongings. Hasan walked into the processing center at about 1:34 in the afternoon. He wore earplugs and pretended to be talking on a cell phone. He told a female civilian at the front desk there was an emergency and the Officer in Charge needed her. The desk had a barrier. Once she left, he yelled "Allah Akbar" and started firing one of his two pistols. He killed 13 and wounded 32 people. Police officers arrived on the scene about 10 minutes later. Officers apprehended Hasan after wounding him (Full Report of Sanity Board, US v MAJ Nidal M Hasan, 13 January 2011. Joshi K, personal communication, July, 2016).[29]

TERRORIST RADICALIZATION ASSESSMENT PROTOCOL-18 INDICATORS
Proximal Warning Behaviors

Pathway

Pathway warning behavior is research, planning, or preparation for an attack, or implementation of an attack.[30,31]

Hasan reportedly spent several days considering the sort of firearm he wanted, inquiring about high-tech weapons at a local weapons retailer, Guns Galore. On August 1, 2009, he bought an FN Five-Seven semiautomatic handgun. Hasan recorded a video of the store manager giving him in-depth usage and care instructions for his new purchase, and he returned nearly every week after to stockpile ammunition. Hasan completed a concealed handgun course on October 10, 2009, and purchased a firing range membership so he could practice there each week.[32] Rather than work on his marksmanship on base, Hasan chose to drive 35 miles to Stan's Outdoor Shooting Range.[29] On the day of the attack, the major wore his fatigues to the processing center, and he filled his cargo pockets with 20 magazines, containing 20 bullets each; he lined the ammunition with paper towels to avoid rattling and attracting suspicion. Lastly, Hasan thought to wear earplugs in preparation for the noise of his attack.[27]

Fixation

Fixation warning behavior indicates an increasingly pathologic preoccupation with a person or a cause, accompanied by a deterioration in social and occupational life.[33]

During his residency, Hasan had become more and more outspoken about his opposition to the military's involvement in Iraq and Afghanistan, proselytizing to classmates, claiming that his religion took precedence over his sworn duties as a serviceman, and even defending suicide bombers. He began fiery arguments about Islam at mosques and alienated himself from more moderate worshipers, friends, and family. Hasan went so far as to express his radical beliefs in class assignments, giving three extraneous, extremist PowerPoint presentations to his superiors and colleagues.[34] Although Hasan graduated from the Virginia Polytechnic Institute and State University with honors and a resume sufficient for acceptance into medical school, his performance as a psychiatric resident and fellow grew markedly worse as his radical beliefs solidified.[29] Both the residency and fellowship programs ranked Hasan in the bottom quarter of his class, and his colleagues regarded him as a slacker and religious zealot. It should be noted that Hasan was accepted into the fellowship program as a placeholder, not for his achievements, for the Army feared losing the fellowship placement when no one else applied. Based on interviews of Hasan's classmates and supervisors, the US Senate[34] reported, "He was placed on probation and remediation and often failed to meet basic job expectations such as showing up for work and being available when he was the physician on call." The same report also concluded that Hasan was a "…barely competent psychiatrist whose radicalization toward violent Islamist extremism alarmed his colleagues and his superiors."[34]

Furthermore, Hasan was an avid reader of extremist materials online, although he particularly favored the radical cleric Anwar al-Awlaki. Awlaki, an American citizen, became a prolific al-Qaeda recruiter, propagandist, and strategist before he was killed in a 2011 US drone strike. Additionally, Hasan, who had never been in a romantic relationship, desperately wanted a marriage that could meet his strict fundamentalist requirements. However, no women were pious enough for him.[27]

Identification

Identification warning behavior indicates a psychological desire to be a pseudocommando,[35,36] have a warrior mentality,[37] closely associate with weapons or other military or law enforcement paraphernalia, identify with previous attackers or assassins, or identify oneself as an agent to advance a particular cause or belief system.[24]

Hasan printed out business cards at some point during his time at Fort Hood (July to November 2009). These made no mention of his military experience, despite his officer status; instead, Hasan identified himself as a "Soldier of Allah" with the abbreviation "SOA" following his name ([27]; first author's files). Along similar lines, Hasan chose silhouette targets over bull's-eye targets during his frequent visits to the firing range.[32] Lastly, Hasan deeply admired other jihadists: Carlos Bledsoe and Awlaki. Just 6 weeks before Hasan's transfer to Fort Hood, Bledsoe attacked a military recruitment center in Little Rock, Arkansas, and Bledsoe's actions stirred Hasan. During his trial, Hasan stated that Bledsoe was "my brother and my friend" (as cited in Ref.[27]).

Novel aggression
Novel aggression warning behavior is an act of violence that seems unrelated to any targeted violence pathway and is committed for the first time.[12] It is typically done to test one's ability to actually be violent. There is no evidence of novel aggression in Hasan's case.

Energy burst
Energy burst warning behavior is an increase in the frequency or variety of any noted activities related to the target, even if the activities themselves are relatively innocuous, usually in the weeks, days, or hours before the attack.[12] Social media activity may increase or decrease during this period of time.

On October 28 and 29, Hasan visited a local strip club, spending nearly 7 hours per night sitting alone by the stage and purchasing several private nude lap dances.[29] Two days before the November 5 massacre, Hasan visited the shooting range and fired more than 200 rounds. He then met with a friend for dinner on November 4th.[28] In the days and hours before he attacked his fellow soldiers, Hasan performed online searches for terms related to the Taliban and jihad.[38]

Leakage
Leakage warning behavior is the communication to a third party of an intent to do harm to a target through an attack.[39]

A fellow Fort Hood psychiatrist testified that Hasan told her a few weeks before the attack that the Army would pay if he were deployed.[38] Furthermore, Hasan endorsed the violent actions of Bledsoe, saying to his fellow Fort Hood officers, "This is what Muslims should do. They should stand up to the aggressor" (as cited in Ref.[27]). Lastly, the major stopped by a convenience store for breakfast about 7 hours before his attack, and he told a customer, "There's going to be a big action on post around 1:30. Be prepared" (as cited in Ref.[29]).

Last resort
Last resort warning behavior is evidence of a "violent action imperative" and/or "time imperative"[40]; it is often a signal of desperation or distress. It is often the result of a triggering event, or one that is anticipated, that involves a loss in love or work.

On October 30, Hasan sent an e-mail to his brother, in which he discussed the following: a resolution to a debt; the power of attorney paperwork he had filled out for his brother; and instructions on handling his affairs should he die or be incapacitated, such as requesting that his brother donate one-third of his wealth to charities as soon as possible after his death.[41] At 2:37 AM on November 5, Hasan called his neighbor; the neighbor did not pick up. He left a message 3 hours later: "Nice knowing you, friend. I'm moving on from here" (as cited in Ref.[29]). Hasan attended 6 AM prayers as he usually did, and he approached a worshipper and apologized for a past slight, before hugging another and explaining he would not be in attendance at the next day's services. On his way home, Hasan stopped in a convenience store, where he made the odd statement about events at the base later that day. In the early hours of daylight, Hasan gave another neighbor frozen broccoli and spinach, an air mattress, and a clothing steamer. He gave away copies of the Koran to other neighbors.[29] Hasan destroyed his birth certificate and medical school degree with a paper shredder before returning to the mosque for noon services; he then drove to the processing center in his combat fatigues.[27] It is important to note that those who witnessed these last resort warning behaviors interpreted them in a specific context: Hasan was about to be deployed to a combat zone.

Directly communicated threat

Directly communicated threat warning behavior is the communication of a direct threat to the target or law enforcement beforehand.[12]

There is no evidence of a directly communicated threat. Hasan made a determined effort to avoid harming noncombatants, using a ruse to send a civilian receptionist in the opposite direction; he targeted soldiers set to deploy, because he believed they posed a threat to his Muslim brothers overseas. Although Hasan did state that the Army would pay if he were to be deployed, he made that statement to a fellow psychiatrist who was not going to be deployed and, therefore, would not endanger Muslims.[27] The psychiatrist was not part of Hasan's target in this situation, so this statement qualifies as leakage only.

Distal Characteristics

Personal grievance and moral outrage

Personal grievance and moral outrage join personal life experience and particular historical, religious, or political events. The personal grievance is often defined by a major loss in love or work, feelings of anger and humiliation, and the blaming of others. Moral outrage is typically a vicarious identification with a group that has suffered, even though the lone-actor terrorist has usually not experienced the same suffering, if any at all.

Hasan experienced some hostility from his fellow soldiers and complained sharply about the general mistreatment of Muslims in the military. In the context of a war sparked from the worst terrorist attack in American history, Hasan felt ostracized by other soldiers. Family members cited three examples of personal affronts: (1) someone had thrown a diaper in his car and told him to use it as a headdress; (2) another had drawn a camel on his car and written "Camel Jockey, Get Out!" underneath; and (3) 3 months before Hasan's attack, a neighbor and veteran scratched Hasan's vehicle with a key in response to his Islamic bumper sticker (personal grievance).[28] Moreover, Hasan claimed in October 2009 that some of his patients had confessed to committing war crimes against Muslims. Hasan was also disgusted by a military he believed to be fighting a war against his religion, and he was even more incensed at the possibility of being involved in that effort once deployed, because his exploration of gaining conscientious objector status had yielded no way out (moral outrage).[34]

Framed by an ideology

Framed by an ideology is the presence of beliefs that justify the terrorist's intent to act. It can be a religious belief system, a political philosophy, a secular commitment, a one-issue conflict, or an idiosyncratic justification.[8,42]

Hasan's mother asked him to explore his faith as her health was declining in 2001, and he became increasingly devout, praying five times a day and attending 4:00 AM prayer services.[27] Around 2004, Hasan began investigating the possibility of leaving the military as a conscientious objector, because he believed a Muslim who killed other Muslims would surely be sent to hell. Two supervisors encouraged his endeavor to leave the Army.[34] Furthermore, Hasan idolized Anwar al-Awlaki and raptly consumed the extremist materials Awlaki shared online. In a series of e-mails to Awlaki, Hasan asked for advice on the issues of Muslims serving in the American military, whether soldiers who committed fratricide for the sake of Islam would be considered martyrs, the appropriateness of killing innocents in the greater service of Islam, the religious legitimacy of suicide bombings with the intention of saving comrades, and several similar topics.[41]

Moreover, Hasan gave three separate extremist PowerPoint presentations from the end of his residency to the end of his fellowship, 2007 to 2008. Supervisory officers, psychiatrists, and other medical professionals comprised the audiences of these presentations. In the first, Hasan discussed the moral ambiguity of Muslims serving in the American military and how this ambiguity led to "adverse events," or incidents of jihadist fratricide within the military. He drew only one conclusion at the end of his presentation: Muslims should be allowed to withdraw as conscientious objectors. The second presentation was so immediately offensive and radical that Hasan's peers objected loudly and the instructor ended the presentation after just 2 minutes; Hasan hypothesized that the US military was at war against Islam, justified suicide bombings, and defended Osama bin Laden. The third presentation connected fratricide and religious conflicts of Muslim soldiers again, but in a slightly more clinical manner: Hasan proposed surveying Muslims in the military about such conflicts. Finally, Hasan shouted "Allahu akbar!" (God is great!) before he shot more than 50 people.[34]

Failure to affiliate with an extremist group
Failure to affiliate with an extremist group is defined by the lone-actor terrorist rejecting or being rejected by a radical or extremist group with which he or she initially wanted to affiliate.

There is no evidence to suggest that Hasan attempted to join a terrorist group or otherwise collaborated with one.

Dependence on the virtual community
Dependence on the virtual community is evidence of the lone-actor terrorist's use of the Internet through social media, chat rooms, e-mails, listservs, texting, tweeting, posting, searches, and so forth concerning his or her radical or extreme beliefs or the planning of tactical operations.

Hasan was active online; he was an ardent consumer of Awlaki's materials, frequenting Awlaki's Web site and subscribing to Awlaki's e-mail service. Hasan sent a total of 18 e-mails to Awlaki from December 2008 to June 2009, yet he received only two messages in reply. He also had Google Alerts for jihadist terms and subscriptions to the following Web sites: Islamicrelief.org, Islamistwatch.org, RadicalIslam.org, and the Middle East Forum.[41]

Thwarting of occupational goals
Thwarting of occupational goals is a major setback or failure in a planned academic and/or occupational life course. According to Hasan's cousin, Nader, combat deployment was Hasan's "worst nightmare" (as cited in Ref.[27]). He admitted to a supervisor that he applied for the fellowship to delay deployment as long as possible, not out of a desire to contribute to his field of study. Furthermore, Hasan wanted to be discharged, but the Army had paid for his medical education, was actively recruiting Arab-Americans, and needed mental health professionals. When he realized achieving

conscientious objector status was not feasible, he resigned himself to completing his Army commitment.[28] When Hasan was transferred to Fort Hood, the Army's staging area for combat deployments at the end of his fellowship, he knew his greatest fear would soon come to fruition. Indeed, the official deployment orders came in October 2009; he was set to embark for Afghanistan at the end of November.[34]

Changes in thinking and emotion

Changes in thinking and emotion is indicated when thoughts and their expression become more strident, simplistic, and absolute. Argument ceases, and preaching begins. Persuasion yields to imposition of one's beliefs on others. There is no critical analysis of theory or opinion, and the mantra, "don't think, just believe," is adopted. Emotions typically move from anger and argument, to contempt and disdain for others' beliefs, to disgust for the outgroup and a willingness to homicidally aggress against them. Violence is cloaked in self-righteousness and the pretense of superior belief. Humor is lost.

This distal characteristic was most apparent from 2001 to 2008. After the successive death of his parents in 1998 and 2001, Hasan became "steadily more pious" and "even more rigid" in his religious views, according to his cousin.[27] Hasan isolated himself from family and friends with accusations of religious failures and engaged in heated arguments about Islam with fellow worshipers, debating the meaning of jihad and the significance of being a true Muslim. Hasan alarmed his peers and superiors inside and outside the classroom; several officers reported him to superiors, and two dubbed him "a ticking time bomb" (as cited in Ref.[34]).

Failure of sexual-intimate pair bonding

Failure of sexual-intimate pair bonding is coded if the subject has historically failed to form a lasting sexually intimate relationship. The sexualization of violence is a secondary component. It refers to the finding of a sexual attitude or behavior in the subject that seems to substitute for the absence of a sexual pair bond, such as the sexualization of weapons, the anticipation of unlimited sexual gratification in the afterlife, the exclusive use of prostitutes and other unbonded sources of sexual gratification, or compulsive use of pornography: all of these behaviors may be rationalized by the ideology. For example, among jihadists, the adoption of Westernized sexual attitudes and behaviors may be acceptable because they help maintain operational secrecy and deceive the unbelievers.

Hasan had never been in a romantic relationship, despite investing a great deal of time and money in finding a mate. He asked several imams to help him find a wife and even attended matchmaking events for single Muslims. But Hasan had high expectations of his future wife: a devout Muslim virgin of Middle Eastern heritage, who prayed five times per day and covered herself appropriately with a hijab. Even when seemingly suitable women expressed an interest in the doctor and officer, they did not meet Hasan's standards. One 2006 event boasted an attendance of 150 single Muslims, yet Hasan complained to the organizer that none of the women appealed to him.[29] He even requested help with romance from Awlaki in a 2008 e-mail.[41] Incongruously, the fundamentalist major began to visit a local strip club in September 2009. He noticed Starz Strip Club after purchasing his handgun next door.[43] Although Hasan's romantic efforts failed terrestrially, he believed his devotion to Islam would be rewarded in the afterlife: in his 2007 residency presentation, Hasan spoke awkwardly about the existence of "a lot of virgins" awaiting the faithful in Paradise (as cited in Ref.[27]).

Mental disorder

Mental disorder is coded if there is evidence of a major mental disorder by history or in the present. Whether or not ideology helps buffer the symptoms of mental disorder is a secondary, but important consideration.[15]

Hasan did not have a diagnosable mental disorder (Full Report of Sanity Board, US v MAJ Nidal M Hasan, 13 January 2011. Joshi K, personal communication, July, 2016).[29]

Greater creativity and innovation

Greater creativity and innovation is coded if there is evidence of tactical thinking "outside the box."[15,42] The planned terrorist act is creative (a major aspect has not been done before in contemporary times) and/or innovative (imitated by others).

Hasan's attack on a US Army base brought about major changes in all branches of the military and several law enforcement agencies, for America had not seen an attack like his before. According to the US Senate,[34] "From September 11th until the Fort Hood attack occurred, the only attack on the homeland that resulted in deaths was perpetrated by a lone-actor Carlos Bledsoe" (p. 19). Representing al Qaeda, US-born Adam Gadahn encouraged others to emulate Hasan's heroic actions in a lengthy video recording of praise: "The Mujahid [one engaged in jihad] brother Nidal Hasan is a pioneer, a trailblazer and a role model who has opened a door, lit a path and shown the way forward for every Muslim who finds himself among the unbelievers and yearns to discharge his duty to Allah and play a part in the defense of Islam and Muslims."[44] Even Awlaki, Hasan's idol, hailed his actions: "I am proud that there are people like Nidal Hasan among my students. ... I support what he did, and I call upon anyone who calls himself a Muslim, and serves in the US army, to follow in the footsteps of Nidal Hasan" (as cited in Ref.[27]).

History of criminal violence

History of criminal violence is coded if there is evidence of instrumental criminal violence in the subject's past. Virtually all acts of terrorism are predatory (instrumental) violence. This characteristic indicates a capacity and a willingness to engage in predation for a variety of reasons, such as a history of armed robberies or planned assaults on others.

No history of criminal violence was found other than the mass murder.

DISCUSSION

Case studies are the idiographic data that put flesh on the bone of large-group nomothetic analyses. Although they typically do not contribute to the advancement of deductive conclusions in science, case studies provide clinicians with a more nuanced and individualized understanding of the application of particular methods to an actual patient. We have applied a structured professional judgment instrument, TRAP-18, to a known outcome case of mass murder, which was clearly ideologically motivated. The results point to a goodness-of-fit between the behaviors of Dr Hasan and the proximal and distal characteristics of the instrument.

What are the practical applications of these findings to a mental health clinician in either a public or private setting? First, it is imperative to note that TRAP-18 does not predict who will or will not commit an act of terrorism. The base rate for such events is extremely low, particularly in the United States, and any attempt at prediction would likely result in a false-positive finding and the potential for deprivation of liberties.

TRAP-18, however, does allow the application of an organized set of indicators that are rationally derived from the lone-actor terrorism research conducted over the past 20 years, and seem to be reliable and have some validity. These indicators can help the clinician determine whether the patient should be monitored for further concerning behavior, or whether the patient should be actively risk managed to divert him or her from a pathway toward ideologically motivated violence. The presence of one warning behavior suggests that the clinical case needs active management (the warning); the presence of only a cluster of distal characteristics suggests that the case needs active monitoring (the watching).[16]

Active risk management could mandate the issuance of a Tarasoff warning, codified in various jurisdictions somewhat differently, but typically requiring the clinician to believe that the patient poses a substantial risk of violence toward an identifiable victim(s), and mandating the notification of the victim and law enforcement. Such decisions on the part of the clinician, however, should be done with the full awareness that federal agencies will be alerted when the term "terrorism" or "terrorist threat" is invoked, and further opportunities to clinically manage the case will probably dissolve. The seriousness of such an action, however, does not preclude its importance when a threat to national security is involved.

Active monitoring, however, calls for a more nuanced approach to a clinical case, including the following:

- Determine if there is a relationship between the patient's diagnosed mental disorder and his or her ideological framing and changes in thinking and emotion. This analysis should be conducted at the level of symptoms rather than diagnosis: is the patient drifting toward a more fundamentalist belief system to modulate his or her anxiety concerning the worsening of symptoms? Is there emerging an esoteric, if not bizarre, belief system that is helping him or her manage a decompensating mind? Is there a causal relationship between certain symptoms and the risk of violence that function as either motivators, disinhibitors, or facilitators?[45] Jared Loughner, the Tucson assassin and mass murderer (but not a terrorist) who wounded Congresswoman Gabrielle Giffords and killed a federal judge in 2011, was diagnosed with schizophrenia, and as he decompensated he embraced nihilism as a philosophy, and the belief that there could be no government if words had no meaning.[12] Theodore Kaczynski, a serial bomber and lone-actor terrorist in the late twentieth century, was diagnosed with paranoid schizophrenia (S. Johnson, psychiatric evaluation, first author's files), and embraced the philosophy of the Luddites, a nineteenth century British textile labor group that raged against advancing technology.
- Therapeutically manage the case with whatever mental health interventions are clinically indicated and feasible. These may include medication adjustments, psychotherapeutic frequency and duration changes, and hospitalization.
- Use collateral contacts with the patient's permission to gather behavioral information concerning the patient's activities when not in treatment, a critical component of a reliable and valid clinical threat assessment using TRAP-18. Families and close friends may be hesitant to provide any information that suggests radicalization for fear of precipitous acts by law enforcement, and dependence on authority figures that have an ongoing relationship with the patient will likely be more informative. It is also imperative that the clinician be aware that family and kinship networks may be supporting the patient's radicalization.[46,47]
- Monitor the patient's online behavior, especially social media activity, by perusing his or her publicly accessible accounts. There is no reasonable expectation of privacy when one posts to Instagram, Facebook, Twitter, and so forth, or any of the other myriad means of expressing oneself in virtual

reality. Clinical threat assessment recognizes that patients increasingly live in terrestrial and virtual reality, and often express their most intimate thoughts and feelings in the latter. Informing the patient of such active monitoring may diminish use of social media; however, it may provide a consensual avenue for more open communication between the mental health professional and the patient.

- Seek consultation with a mental health professional that is of the same racial, ethnic, or religious background of the patient so cultural behaviors are not grossly misinterpreted by the treating clinician.

SUMMARY

The violence of the lone-actor terrorist cannot be predicted; however, in many cases, it can be prevented. In this article we have studied the behaviors and mindset of a lone-actor terrorist, Malik Hasan (who happened to also be a mental health professional and a psychiatrist) through the lens of TRAP-18. Trained clinicians observed his behaviors for years, yet he continued on a pathway to targeted violence, culminating in the worst act of domestic terrorism in the United States since 9/11. Such acts are very low-frequency, but high-intensity events. They are understandable, and interdiction is possible. The fictional writer in the novel *Mao II*[48] ruefully noted, "Years ago I used to think it was possible for a novelist to alter the inner life of the culture. Now bomb-makers and gunmen have taken that territory. They make raids on human consciousness." Mental health clinicians are uniquely qualified and positioned to carefully observe such consciousness when it turns homicidally dark; they may therapeutically divert, and in some cases, operationally intervene with law enforcement to mitigate the risks of such mobilization for targeted violence.

REFERENCES

1. Meloy JR. The empirical basis and forensic application of affective and predatory violence. Australian and New Zealand J. Psychiatry 2006;40:539–47.

2. Meloy JR. Approaching and attacking public figures: a contemporary analysis of communications and behavior. In: Chauvin C, editor. Threatening communications and behavior: perspectives on the pursuit of public figures. Board on Behavioral, Cognitive, and Sensory sciences, Division of Behavioral and Social Sciences and Education. Washington, DC: The National Academies Press; 2011. p. 75–101.

3. Monahan J. The individual risk of terrorism. Psychol Public Pol L 2012;18: 167–205.

4. McEllistrem J. Affective and predatory violence: a bimodal classification system of human aggression and violence. Aggression Violent Behav 2004;10:1–30.

5. Meloy JR, Hoffmann J, editors. International handbook of threat assessment. New York: Oxford Univ. Press; 2014.

6. Fein R, Vossekuil B, Holden G. Threat assessment: an approach to prevent targeted violence. NCJ Publication 155000. Washington, DC: U.S. Dept. of Justice; Office of Justice Programs; National Institute of Justice; 1995.

7. Fein R, Vossekuil B. Preventing attacks on public officials and public figures: A Secret Service Perspective. In: Meloy JR, editor. The psychology of Stalking: clinical and forensic perspectives. San Diego, CA: Academic Press; 1998. p. 176–91.

8. Meloy JR, Hart S, Hoffmann J. Threat assessment and threat management. In: Meloy JR, Hoffmann J, editors. International handbook of threat assessment. New York: Oxford Univ. Press; 2014. p. 3–17.

9. Monahan J. The individual risk assessment of terrorism: recent developments. In: LaFree G, Freilich J, editors. The handbook of the criminology of terrorism. Hoboken (NJ): John Wiley and Sons; 2016.

10. Meloy, JR. (2011). Violent true believers. FBI Law Enforcement Bulletin (July). Available at: www.leb.fbi.gov. Accessed March 15, 2016.

11. Meloy, JR. (2016). Identifying warning behaviors of the individual terrorist. FBI Law Enforcement Bulletin (April). Available at: www.leb.fbi.gov. Accessed May 7, 2016.

12. Meloy JR, Hoffmann J, Guldimann A, et al. The role of warning behaviors in threat assessment: an exploration and suggested typology. Behav Sci L 2012;30: 256–79.

13. Siegel A, Victoroff J. Understanding human aggression: new insights from neuroscience. Int J L Psychiatry 2009;32:209–15.

14. Meloy JR. Indirect assessment of the violent true believer. J Personal Assess 2004;82:138–46.

15. Meloy JR, Yakeley J. The violent true believer as a "lone wolf": psychoanalytic perspectives on terrorism. Behav Sci L 2014;32:347–65.

16. Monahan J, Steadman H. Violent storms and violent people. Am Psychol 1996;51: 931–8.

17. Hoffmann J, Meloy JR, Guldimann A, et al. Attacks on German public figures, 1968-2004: warning behaviors, potentially lethal and nonlethal acts, psychiatric status, and motivations. Behav Sci L 2011;29:155–79.

18. Hoffmann J, Glaz-Ocik J, Roshdi K et al. Terrorismus und Anschläge durch radikalisierte Einzeltäter. In: Hoffmann J, Roshdi K, editors. Amok und andere Formen schwerer Gewalt: Risikoanalyse - Bedrohungsmanagement - Präventionskonzepte. Stuttgart (Germany): Schattauer; p. 244–265, in press.

19. Meloy JR, Hoffmann J, Roshdi K, et al. Some warning behaviors discriminate between school shooters and other students of concern. J Threat Assess Management 2014;1:203–11.

20. Meloy JR, Roshdi K, Glaz-Ocik J, et al. Investigating the individual terrorist in Europe. J Threat Assess Management 2015;2:140–52.

21. Bockler N, Hoffmann J, Zick A. The Frankfurt Airport attack: a case study on the radicalization of a lone actor terrorist. J Threat Assess Management 2015;2: 153–63.

22. Meloy JR, Habermeyer E, Guldimann A. The warning behaviors of Anders Breivik. J Threat Assess Management 2015;2:164–75.

23. Meloy JR, Hoffmann J, Roshdi K, et al. Warning behaviors and their configurations across various domains of targeted violence. In: Meloy JR, Hoffmann J, editors. International handbook of threat assessment. New York: Oxford University Press; 2014a. p. 39–53.

24. Meloy JR, Gill P. The lone actor terrorist and the TRAP-18. J Threat Assess Management 2016;3:37–52.

25. Meloy JR, Mohandie K, Knoll J, et al. The concept of identification in threat assessment. Behav Sci L 2015;33:213–37.

26. New America Foundation. 2016. Available at: http://securitydata.newamerica.net/extremists/deadly-attacks.html. Accessed August 2, 2016.

27. Bergen P. The United States of jihad: investigating America's homegrown terrorists. New York: Crown Publishers; 2016.

28. McKinley J, Dao J. Fort Hood gunman gave signals before his rampage. The New York Times 2009. Available at: http://www.nytimes.com.
29. Saslow E, Rucker P, Wan W, et al. In aftermath of Fort Hood, community haunted by clues that went unheeded. The Washington Post 2009. Available at: http://www.washingtonpost.com.
30. Calhoun F, Weston S. Contemporary threat management. San Diego (CA): Specialized Training Services; 2003.
31. Fein R, Vossekuil B. Assassination in the United States: an operational study of recent assassins, attackers, and near lethal approachers. J Forensic Sci 1999; 44:321–33.
32. Brown AK, Graczyk M. Hasan repeatedly visited firing range before Fort Hood rampage. The Washington Post 2010. Available at: http://www.washingtonpost.com.
33. Mullen P, James D, Meloy JR, et al. The fixated and the pursuit of public figures. J Forensic Psychiatry and Psychology 2009;20:33–47.
34. U.S. Senate Committee on Homeland Security and Governmental Affairs. A ticking time bomb: counterterrorism lessons from the U.S. government's failure to prevent the Fort Hood Attack. 2011. Available at: http://www.hsgac.senate.gov. Accessed July 18, 2016.
35. Dietz P, Martell D. Mentally disordered offenders in pursuit of celebrities and politicians. Washington, DC: Institute of Justice; 1989.
36. Knoll J. The "pseudocommando" mass murderer: Part I, the psychology of revenge and obliteration. J Am Acad Psychiatry Law 2010;38:87–94.
37. Hempel A, Meloy JR, Richards T. Offender and offense characteristics of a nonrandom sample of mass murderers. J Am Acad Psychiatry and the Law 1999;27:213–25.
38. Fernandez M. Fort Hood gunman told his superiors of concerns. The New York Times 2013. Available at: http://www.nytimes.com.
39. Meloy JR, ÓToole ME. The concept of leakage in threat assessment. Behav Sci L 2011;29:513–27.
40. Mohandie, K & Duffy, J. (1999). First responder and negotiation guidelines with the paranoid schizophrenic subject. FBI Law Enforcement Bulletin, 8–16. Available at: Leb.fbi.gov. Accessed April 19, 2016.
41. Federal Bureau of Investigation. Final report of the William H. Webster commission on the Federal Bureau of Investigation, counterterrorism intelligence, and the events at Fort Hood, Texas, on November 5, 2009. 2012. Available at: https://www.fbi.gov. Accessed November 2, 2015.
42. Simon J. Lone wolf terrorism: understanding the growing threat. Amherst (NY): Prometheus Books; 2013.
43. Shane S, Dao J. Investigators study tangle of clues on Fort Hood suspect. The New York Times 2009. Available at: http://www.nytimes.com.
44. Verjee, Z. 2010. Report of American al Qaeda spokesman's arrest questioned. Cable News Network. Available at: http://www.cnn.com. Accessed March 1, 2016.
45. Douglas K, Guy L, Hart S. Psychosis and violence. Psychol Bull 2009;135(5): 679–706.
46. Gill P. Lone-actor terrorists. New York: Routledge; 2015.
47. Guldimann A, Hoffmann J, Meloy JR. Eine Einführung in die Warnverhalten Typologie. In: Hoffmann J, Roshdi K, editors. Bedrohungsmanagement – Projekte und Erfahrungen aus der Schweiz. Frankfurt/Main (Germany): Verlag für Polizeiwissenschaft; 2013.
48. DeLillo D. Mao II. New York: Penguin Group; 1992.

Stalking and Violence

Britta Ostermeyer, MD, MBA[a],*, Susan Hatters Friedman, MD[b],
Renee Sorrentino, MD[c], Brad D. Booth, MD, FRCPC[d]

KEYWORDS

- Violence • Stalking • Classification • Women • Juveniles • Health care providers
- Violence risk assessment • Risk management

KEY POINTS

- There are three well recognized stalker classification systems: Zona and colleagues' Stalker-Victim Types; Mullen and colleagues' Stalker Typology; and the RECON Stalker Typology.
- In female stalkers, the violence risk should be taken seriously. Given their high rates of mental illness and personality disorder, women stalkers should undergo psychiatric examinations.
- Juvenile stalking can also be associated with violence, and risk should be considered.
- Clinicians may be stalked and can become a victim of a special type of stalking behavior, referred to as stalking by proxy.
- Threats and violence are common in stalking. Evaluation of risk factors allows for a violence risk-reduction plan, which can guide stalking intervention.

STALKER CLASSIFICATIONS

Stalking refers to a constellation of repeated and persistent behaviors to impose unwanted communication and/or contact on another person.[1,2] Communication can be via telephone calls, text, e-mails, letters, paper notes, or graffiti writings. Unwanted contact can be by approaching and/or following the victim; maintaining surveillance; appearing in places the victim is expected; and/or visiting the victim's home, family, and/or friends. Additional behaviors may include ordering goods or canceling appointments on the victim's behalf or initiating bogus legal actions. Threats, property damage, and/or physical assaults may accompany stalking.[1,2] Stalking behavior can provide helpful insights about the stalkers themselves. Men are more likely than

Disclosures: The authors have nothing to disclose.
[a] Department of Psychiatry and Behavioral Sciences, University of Oklahoma, 920 Stanton L. Young Boulevard, #WP3470, Oklahoma City, OK 73104, USA; [b] Department of Psychological Medicine, University of Auckland, Auckland Hospital Support Building, Room 12-003, Grafton, Auckland, New Zealand; [c] Department of Psychiatry, Harvard School of Medicine, 15 Parkman Street, Boston, MA 02114, USA; [d] Department of Psychiatry, University of Ottawa, 2nd Floor – Forensics, 1145 Carling Avenue, Ottawa, Ontario K1Z 7K4, Canada
* Corresponding author.
E-mail address: britta-ostermeyer@ouhsc.edu

Psychiatr Clin N Am 39 (2016) 663–673
http://dx.doi.org/10.1016/j.psc.2016.07.010
0193-953X/16/© 2016 Elsevier Inc. All rights reserved.
psych.theclinics.com

women to use stalking as a means of continuing to control and intimidate their ex-partner.[3]

Most studies have focused on male stalkers because close to 80% of stalking is done by men.[1–3] However, the lifetime risk of being stalked is 8% for women and 2% for men.[1]

Although there is no consensus in the forensic or psychiatric community on a single stalker classification system,[4] there are three recognized stalker classifications: (1) Zona and colleagues'[5] Stalker-Victim Types, (2) Mullen and colleagues'[1,2] Stalker Typology, and (3) The RECON (RElationship and CONtext-Based) Stalker Typology.[6]

These three typology classifications studied only adult stalkers. Although they may have some validity in juveniles, juveniles were not evaluated in these studies. These stalker classifications were created with the goals of identifying differences among groups of stalkers to develop helpful management and treatment recommendations and to improve violence risk predictions. Published stalker classifications focus on the stalker's relationship with the victim and on the degree to which violence was an issue.[4]

Based on violence risk prediction, Zona and colleagues'[5] Stalker-Victim typology described three types of stalkers: (1) simple obsessionals, (2) love obsessionals, and (3) erotomanics. This typology was derived from the Los Angeles Police Department's Threat Management Unit. The largest group of the simple obsessionals usually has a prior relationship with victims, make more physical contact, and carry a high risk of violence; the erotomanics are the rarest Zona group, usually with less contact with victims, and a lower risk of violence.[5]

The Mullen and colleagues'[1,2] Stalker Typology originated at an Australian forensic center and expanded the prior classification to include motivation for the stalking. It described five stalker types that are not mutually exclusive: (1) the rejected, (2) the intimacy seekers, (3) the incompetent, (4) the resentful, and (5) the predatory.[1,2] The rejected stalkers are usually disgruntled ex-intimates with the highest risk for assaults and with initial highly ambivalent motives of reconciliation and revenge. Such stalkers replace the lost relationship with the victim with their stalking behaviors. The resentful and predatory stalkers also carry a higher risk of violence. Whereas the resentful stalker feels wronged by the victim, the often sadistic predatory stalker prepares for a violent and/or sexual attack onto the victim. The intimacy seekers are the most persistent of all stalkers in their stalking, at times stalking for years or even decades.[1,2]

The RECON Stalker Typology is based on the nature and the context of the stalker-victim relationship and its violence risk prediction.[6] This latest typology, derived from a study of 1005 North Americans by Mohandie and colleagues,[6] separated stalkers into two main types based on whether or not the stalker and victim had a prior relationship or not. Then, each type is further subdivided into two subtypes of stalkers based on the context of the stalker-victim relationship[6]:

- Type I, prior relationship
  - A. Intimate stalker
  - B. Acquaintance stalker
- Type II, no prior relationship
  - A. Public figure stalker
  - B. Private stranger

The intimate stalkers, which were the largest group, were most violent and malignant with 83% who threatened violence and almost three-quarters (74%) who were actually violent. They were usually male, with a prior criminal history, and with high recidivism despite a protective order or incarceration. Acquaintance stalkers were more likely to be psychotic at the time of an offense and less likely to reoffend than the intimate stalker, but two-thirds (66%) of the acquaintance stalkers made threats and half (50%) were violent. Although public figure stalkers were the least likely to be violent, private stranger stalkers showed that half (50%) threatened and 36% were violent.

FEMALE STALKERS

When men report being stalked, they may experience indifference, or may be told they should be flattered. Women are rarely prosecuted for stalking. Women may stalk men, or may stalk other women. In fact, women are more likely to engage in same-gender stalking than are men.[7]

Women often have similar motivations as men for stalking.[7] However, female stalkers are more likely to be trying to establish an intimate relationship, whereas male stalkers are more likely to be trying to maintain an intimate relationship.[8] Female stalkers are more likely than male stalkers to stalk professional contacts, including psychiatrists. Like their male counterparts, they are most likely to be violent toward former intimates who they stalk. Borderline personality disorder and erotomania are more commonly found among female stalkers.[7]

Rates of female stalkers vary depending on the sample type, ranging from approximately 1 in 10 stalkers being female to one in four stalkers.[9] An American community study found 12% to 13% of stalkers were women[10]; whereas an Australian forensic team specializing in stalking found 21%.[11]

Purcell and colleagues[11] reviewed 40 female cases referred to a forensic stalking team. Most were not in stable relationships, although most were employed. One-half had a personality disorder and approximately one-third (30%) had a delusional disorder. Most stalked someone they knew; 40% of the victims were professional contacts. Approximately half stalked other women, and half stalked men, with a similar tenacity as male stalkers. Regarding motive as described by Mullen and colleagues,[1,2] intimacy seekers were most common, followed by rejected stalkers, resentful stalkers, and finally incompetent stalkers. Similarly to men, one-half threatened violence, approximately one-quarter (23%) assaulted, and one-third engaged in property damage. Women were less likely than men to have a history of arrests (18% vs 43%), have a history of violent offenses (13% vs 31%), abuse substances (8% vs 28%), stalk a stranger (5% vs 21%), or follow their victim (50% vs 78%).[11] Women were more likely than men to call their victims (98% vs 73%), stalk a professional contact (40% vs 17%), have a victim of the same gender (48% vs 9%), and to have an intimacy-seeking motive (45% vs 29%).[11]

Meloy and Boyd[12] surveyed stalking experts in North America and Australia about their cases of female stalkers. Of their 82 cases, the mean age was in the late 30s. One-third were mothers. Two-thirds of the victims were males. Most had graduated high school, and 38% had a college degree. When the IQ was known, it was average to superior. Approximately one-half had psychotic disorders, one-third had been psychiatrically admitted, and one-third were using substances. Many had experienced abuse. In the year before the stalking, these women had commonly experienced a significant loss. Borderline personality disorder, with its intensity of attachment, instability, and underlying fear of abandonment, was the most common personality disorder. More than one-third had a criminal history. Regarding whom they stalked, one-half stalked prior acquaintances, 27% stalked prior intimates, and 21% stalked strangers. Regarding methods of stalking, one-half followed their victims, most sent letters and unwanted gifts, and made telephone calls.[12]

Although 65% threatened their victims, 25% were actually physically violent. Threats were noted to be either expressive or instrumental (to control the victim's behavior). Weapons used were a knife, gun, or car, but injury did not usually require medical attention. Meloy and Boyd[12] noted that violence was usually affective, although homicides were predatory.

Similarly, Meloy and colleagues[13] using law enforcement, prosecutorial, and entertainment corporate security files, reviewed 143 female stalker cases, finding similarly that female stalkers, on average, were unpartnered and in their mid-30s with a psychiatric diagnosis. Regarding risk, they found "The most dangerous subgroup was the prior sexually intimate stalkers, of whom the majority both threatened and were physically violent. The least dangerous were the female stalkers of the Hollywood celebrities."[13]

Finally, Strand and McEwan[14] combined a Swedish police sample and an Australian specialist stalking clinic sample. Most women stalked someone known to them, including prior intimates. The most frequent motive was rejected stalker, followed by resentful stalkers and intimacy seekers. Women were more likely than men to have borderline personality disorder (33% vs 2%), and had a trend of being more likely to be psychotic (38% vs 20%).[14] Although men were more likely to follow their victims, women were more likely to stalk by e-mail or letter. Almost one-quarter of the female stalkers were violent (23%). The women who were violent were more likely to be using substances, be stalking a former sexual partner, and to have a rejected stalker motivation. Critically, Strand and McEwan[14] found that for both gender stalkers, there was an 80% chance of violence if they possessed the following three characteristics: (1) prior intimate relationship, (2) approach behavior, and (3) making threats.

JUVENILE STALKERS

Until recently, juvenile stalking was thought to be rare and therefore not studied.[15] The absence of studies on juvenile stalkers may be explained by the tendency to view juveniles as incapable of stalking, and to interpret what may seem to be stalking-like behaviors as a part of developmental phases. For example, grade school boys and girls often develop an idealized love interest, such as a celebrity or the most popular student in the school. As part of this idealized love interest or "crush" the boy or girl may send multiple electronic communications, texts, or gifts to demonstrate their interest. The juvenile may follow the love interest or make attempts to learn where the love interest lives. These behaviors have traditionally been considered appropriate to the juvenile's developmental age. However, emerging evidence suggests some juveniles engage in the behaviors described in adult stalkers. Stalking should be distinguished from bullying. The definition of bullying varies, but in general refers to when an individual is threatened, humiliated, or harassed by another individual. The main intention of bullying is to socially isolate the victim. The distinction between stalking and bullying is not always clear. Some studies have distinguished bullying from stalking based on where the behaviors occur. Purcell and colleagues[16] suggest that stalking, unlike bullying, involves forcing oneself on the attentions of another in a context where you have no legitimate right to be. Although the prevalence of juvenile stalking is unknown, studies have confirmed the presence of juvenile stalkers and begun to identify characteristics associated with perpetrators and victims.

McCann's[17] research of 13 obsessional followers shows the reality of juvenile stalkers. The study, although small, found interesting results about stalking behaviors among juveniles. It reported that juvenile stalkers, like adult stalkers, tend to be mostly male with female victims, who may use threats (about one-half) and violence (about one-third).[17] The primary motivation for stalking in McCann's study was the desire for sexual contact.[17]

Purcell and colleagues[16] more recently published an empirical study about the extent, nature, and impact of juvenile stalking. The study of 299 juvenile stalkers identified some important differences when compared with adult stalkers.[16] Although most juvenile stalkers were males (64%) stalking female victims (69%), there were relatively more female juvenile stalkers than in the adult population studies. Nearly all of the juvenile stalkers stalked a previously known victim (98%). Overall, more than half (57%) involved same-gender stalking, with females more likely (86%) than males (40%) pursuing same gender victims. The most common modalities of stalking were approaching the victim, telephoning the victim, or sending text messages. Three-fourths (75%) of the victims were threatened. One-half (54%) of victims were physically assaulted (ranging from cuts and bruises to serious injuries). When compared with adult stalkers, fewer cases of juvenile stalkers were motivated by the desire to initiate a relationship or date the victim and a larger portion was motivated by retaliation and antisocial behaviors. Like adult stalkers, juvenile stalkers were motivated by rejection, the pursuit of intimacy, and predation.[16]

In a follow-up study, Purcell and colleagues[18] examined gender differences in juvenile stalkers. Male juvenile stalkers were more likely to stalk prior intimates when compared with female juvenile offenders who were more likely to stalk estranged friends. Same-gender stalking was more common in females. Additionally, Purcell and colleagues[18] discovered gender differences for stalking motivation: male juvenile stalkers were more likely motivated by rejection and sexual predation when compared with female stalkers, who were more likely motivated by bullying and retaliation. However, McCann's[17] study found sexual interest to be the primary stalking motivation.

Although there has not been an empirically studied classification for juvenile stalkers, Evans and Meloy[15] formulated a juvenile stalker classification based on two case studies. The typology is comprised by type I, socially awkward; and type 2, angry or disgruntled. They postulated that the angry or disgruntled group posed a higher risk of violence. However, this typology has not been sufficiently studied.

Purcell and colleagues[16] classified stalkers into six classifications:

1. Stalking as an extension of bullying
2. Retaliating stalkers
3. Rejected stalkers
4. Disorganized and disturbed stalkers
5. Predatory stalkers
6. Intimacy-seeking stalkers

They found the most common motivations to be retaliation, rejection, and stalking as an extension of bullying.

STALKING OF MENTAL HEALTH PROFESSIONALS

Mental health professionals are at times requested to assist those who are victims of stalking. However, mental health professionals are not immune to becoming a victim of stalking.

The rates of stalking of mental health professionals are variable. McIvor and colleagues[19] reported that in a large mental health organization, 21% of psychiatrists had been stalked. The length of stalking lasted from weeks to years. In an Irish study, 25% of psychiatrists reported being stalked; actual rates may be higher.[20] In a large-scale study of UK psychiatrists, 21% reported being stalked.[21] However, 31%

reported experiencing behaviors directed toward them that would legally be classified as stalking, suggesting mental health professionals may tend to minimize these issues.

The types of stalking behaviors that mental health professionals are exposed to can include receiving unwanted telephone calls, letters, and approaches; receiving personal threats; and being followed, spied on, or subject to surveillance.[22] However, clinicians can also become victims of a special type of stalking behavior, referred to as stalking by proxy.[2,23] In this form of stalking, the stalker may start by using traditional stalking methods of calls, letters, surveillance, and other unwanted contact. However, the stalker then enlists unbiased third parties with complaints against the clinician. This may include the psychiatrist's hospital administration, licensing bodies, police, media, human rights tribunals, colleagues, civil courts, and others. These third parties are unaware of the stalker's history, and thus naively take up the cause of the stalker, acting as a proxy for the stalker. The third parties embark on repeated contact with the psychiatrist under the assumption that the stalker's complaints may have merit. This can result in repeated reawakening of the stalking; as one lengthy complaint is resolved, other complaints replace this resulting in months or years of emotional stress, professional stress, spent time, and financial tolls on the clinician-victim. Although ultimately the complaints are frivolous and vexatious, the cost to the psychiatrist is the same.

More rarely, stalking of clinicians can escalate beyond harassing behaviors and can include serious physical violence.[24] Mastronardi and colleagues[25] noted up to 20% of stalked psychiatrists were physically assaulted. Outside of physical harm, clinicians may experience anxiety, sleep disturbance, anhedonia, and low motivation from stalking.[21] They may also have concern for the safety of their family.

When faced with stalking, 25% of clinicians do not seek any assistance.[21] This highlights the need for awareness and support of colleagues who may be facing this stress.[26]

VIOLENCE RISK ASSESSMENT AND RISK MANAGEMENT

Threats and violent behaviors in stalking are not uncommon. Reports show that stalkers make threats in about half of the cases, and physical violence occurs in about a third of the cases, with infrequent serious physical injury.[1–3] Physical violence is usually limited to assault and battery, such as punching and grabbing without a weapon. When weapons are used, stalkers usually intend to intimidate and control victims rather than physically injure them.[3] Although threats are common and are associated with violence in stalking, violence can also occur without prior threats, and threats may not go on to violence.[2,3]

General risk factors for violence by stalkers include substance abuse, making threats, suicidality of the stalker, and a prior intimate relationship with the victim.[3] There is a consensus that victims who had a prior intimate relationship with their stalker are at a higher risk of physical violence.[2,3] Ex-intimates were the most likely to be physically harmed, followed by estranged relatives or previous friends, and then followed by casual acquaintances, work-related people, and lastly, strangers.[2] The more intimate the relationship between the stalker and the victim, the more likely a threat would be carried out.[3] The more specific the threat, the more likely it is carried out.[27] Threats made in person face to face are more likely to be carried out than those made on the telephone or in writing.[27] In fewer than 20% of cases, the stalker becomes violent toward third parties, usually those perceived by the stalker to impede access to the victim, such as a current partner.[3,28] Property damage occurs at about half of the rate of personal violence, with the victim's car being the most often vandalized object. Homes were also frequently targeted.[2,3,28]

Studies show that the most significant predictor for major violence was a prior sexual relationship.[3,24] In particular, psychological abuse during the relationship was the strongest predictor of subsequent stalking of a serious and potentially dangerous type.[3,29] James and Farnham[24] found that the risk factors for severe violence and homicide by stalkers included prior history of violence, appearing at the victim's home, leaving threatening messages on the victim's car, threats to harm the victim's children, and major depression in the stalker.

Substance abuse increases the violence risk because it can impair impulse control, increase emotions including anger, and lead to paranoid thinking, which can lead to more aggressive behaviors.[30]

Mohandie and colleagues[6] attempted to simplify the violence risk evaluation process by placing stalkers into risk categories by using prior relationship as the sole variable[2]: High risk (ex-intimates), medium risk (acquaintances, strangers with direct contact), and low risk (strangers without prior direct access to victim). Purcell and colleagues[31] also found that stalking-related violence varied according to prior relationship: ex-intimates had a high risk of violence, acquaintances and strangers who have been in direct contact had a medium risk, and strangers without any prior relationship to the victim had a low risk. Although this simple process enables separating stalkers into large risk groups, it is inadequate by itself given that about 50% of ex-partners and 10% of strangers attack.[2]

Interestingly, psychotic stalkers are less likely to be physically violent than their nonpsychotic counterparts.[2] Although Mullen and colleagues[2] report that the evidence for an association between past criminal or violent behavior and stalking violence is inconsistent, they encourage to not abandon these variables in any risk assessment until the relationship is clarified.[2]

When evaluating the stalking of a health care professional, it is important to seek the assistance of an unbiased third party or unbiased colleague because the ability to assess risk by the victim health care professional can be compromised.

Mullen and colleagues[2] urge mental health professionals to gain some picture of the likely stalking progress and to identify factors in which modification may improve the outcome. Mullen and colleagues[2] propose evaluation of the following domains:

1. The nature of the relationship between the stalker and the victim
2. The stalker's motivations
3. The psychological, psychopathological, and social realities of the stalker
4. The psychological and social vulnerabilities of the victim
5. The legal and mental health context in which the stalking is occurring

Rejected ex-intimates are most likely to assault.[2] Most of their attacks are not serious physical injuries; however, a good number inflict serious or even fatal injuries.[2] In particular, in the process of leaving the relationship, a victim is at high risk of assault. Although stalkers of celebrities and public figures rarely attack, they often intend to inflict serious or lethal injuries when they do.[2]

When it comes to stalking duration, Purcell and colleagues[32] found in an empirical study that either stalkers subsided at 2 weeks or less or they move on to stalking for more than 6 months and longer. Those who stalked for up to 2 weeks usually stalked strangers, whereas those who stalked for long durations usually knew their victims before the stalking.

Rosenfeld[33] found that about half (49%) of stalkers reoffend in a longitudinal study, 80% of whom reoffended during the first year. The strongest predictors of recidivism included the presence of a personality disorder, and in particular, a "Cluster B" personality disorder (ie, antisocial, borderline, and/or narcissistic). Those offenders with both a personality disorder and a history of substance abuse were significantly more likely to reoffend compared with either of these risk factors alone.[33] Interestingly, delusional stalkers had a lower reoffending risk,[33] and perhaps more aggressive psychiatric treatment in those psychotic stalkers explains this finding.[3] Factors, such as shared work or custody, which reinforce contact between the stalker and victim, predispose to stalking recurrence.[2]

Often victims do not report the stalking because of fears of escalation to violence by the stalkers and concerns that police will not do anything to stop the stalking. Indeed, discouraging the stalking behaviors may increase stalking behaviors and the violence risk.[3]

When mental health professionals evaluate stalking, it is recommended to use a multidisciplinary team approach, comprised of the victim, mental health experts, police, the prosecutor, and security specialists.[3] At first, the team needs to establish that stalking indeed is taking place to rule out false victimization claims. This requires essential access to collateral information, such as police records, witness statements, victim impact reports, judges' sentencing remarks, and, if available, prior mental health records of the victim and the stalker. Next, interviews of the victim, police, other witnesses, and, if possible, the stalker should be conducted.

Once the stalking is substantiated, the ultimate need is for advice and guidance by the team about what should be done to reduce or avoid damaging outcomes.[2] A periodic risk assessment is often necessary because of stalking's chronic nature and the stalker's potential behavioral changes depending on given situations.[2] Risk in stalking depends on interactions and can change as situations change. These changes in interactions and situation may allow for a risk-reduction intervention.[2] By viewing the situation through the stalker's eyes, the team needs to carefully ascertain whether a certain intervention would escalate the stalker's conduct or would get the stalker to retreat from the stalking behavior.[2,34] Interventions that potentially humiliate the stalker are of particular concern, because then the stalker is at higher risk of acting out violently.[2]

Violence toward former intimate partners is usually affective in nature, that is, highly emotional, impulsive, and unplanned.[3,35] In contrast, violence toward public figures is likely predatory, with cool emotions, goal directed, and planned.[3,35] In public figure stalking, stalkers usually do not communicate prior threats before an intended violent act, because such prior communication would lessen their chance of success.[3] Hence, related to violence risk prediction, it is helpful to figure out what type of violence the stalker is likely to use.[3]

When evaluating a stalker, the evaluator needs to gather a full history of the stalker's past relationships, past stalking behaviors, current relationships, and current stalking behaviors, such as how much time and resources are spent on current behaviors, and how much time is spent thinking about the victim. Also, the evaluator should seek to understand the stalker's reasoning and objectives for the current stalking; should seek to review prior and current police and psychiatric records; and may interview the stalker's family, friends, neighbors, employers, or teachers.

A violence risk assessment is more than an identification of the risk factors. It is important to evaluate the likelihood, the seriousness/magnitude, occurrence/recurrence, and imminence of a violent event.[2] These aspects cannot simply be added up, because there are often tradeoffs between the components. A potentially imminent but less serious event might be of more importance than a serious but unlikely and distant event. In addition, one should identify the factors that can increase the likelihood of a violent event in a particular stalker and identify factors that are potentially modifiable by intervention.[2] Mullen and colleagues[2] advise to first place the stalker into a group with a known level of risk (see stalker classifications) and then identify risk factors. Those factors that can be modified to decrease the risk should then be identified in a process of moving from stalker group attributes to individual stalker solutions.

Risk factors for violence can be classified into static or dynamic.[36] Static risk factors are not subject to change by intervention (eg, historical information, such as demographics and past history). By looking at the static risk factors, one can place the stalker into a group with high, medium, or low risk of violence.[2] However, dynamic risk factors are subject to change by intervention, such as living situation, psychotic symptoms, medication noncompliance, or access to weapons.[36] As part of a violence risk assessment, one should compose a violence risk-reduction plan.[36] In such a plan, which may be in table format, each dynamic risk factor is listed (column A) with the planned intervention to successfully address that risk factor (column B) alongside a current status update on each risk factor/intervention plan scenario (column C). An example of such a risk reduction plan is illustrated in **Table 1**.

Restraining orders or protective injunctions against stalkers are contentious.[2] Although they may deter some stalkers from stalking, there is a high rate of violation.[2,3] They work best in stalkers with limited emotional attachment and are likely to be ineffective against former intimates with significant emotional investment and preoccupation with the victim. Additionally, they are usually ineffective in delusional or erotomanic stalkers with an unreal understanding of the relationship. It is important not to have a false sense of security from such orders because they can only be enforced once breached.[3]

The general approach to the evaluation of a juvenile stalker is not unlike the approach to adults. The assessment is based on the data gleaned from adult stalkers because little is known about juvenile stalkers. An evaluation should first determine if stalking occurred. Bullying, sexual harassment, and dating violence can be associated with stalking and maybe mistaken as such. Next, a comprehensive psychiatric history should be obtained including the presence of violence, threats, previous stalking behavior, and other stalking behaviors.

Although the evaluation is based on risk assessment variables borrowed from the adult stalking literature, attention should be paid to the developmental phase of the juvenile stalker. This includes understanding the stalker's relationship with peers, influence of others, role of parental figures, and the stalker's emotional maturity. Also, the manner in which the juvenile committed the stalking behavior should be explored (social media, texting, telephone records, e-mails) because it may yield valued insight into the stalking behavior.

The psychiatric assessment of a juvenile stalker should also determine if a major mental illness is associated with the stalking behavior. Although the prevalence of

Table 1
Violence prevention plan example

Risk Factors	Management/Treatment	Status
1. Victim in contact with stalker	1. Victim to cease all contact	1. Completed
2. Victim provokes stalker	2. Victim to cease, counseling for victim	2. Initiated
3. Depression in stalker	3. Antidepressant, psychotherapy for stalker	3. Initiated
4. Substance abuse in stalker	4. Substance abuse treatment for stalker	4. Pending

psychosis in juvenile stalkers is unknown, the presence of psychosis has important treatment implications. Collateral data from family, peers, and victims should be obtained. A general violence risk assessment should be conducted in the same manner as in adult stalking.

SUMMARY

There are adult stalker classifications that can aid the stalking risk assessment. Although most stalking is by men, women and juveniles are also known to stalk and pose violence risk to their victims. Stalking of health care professionals may have particular concerns, such as "stalking by proxy." Although it is important to ascertain static and dynamic violence risk factors in a stalking risk assessment, the dynamic risk factors may offer opportunity for intervention and management of the stalking. It is the goal of any stalking intervention to lower the violence risk and facilitate best possible outcomes.

REFERENCES

1. Mullen PE, Pathé M, Purcell R, et al. Study of stalkers. Am J Psychiatry 1999;56: 1244–9.
2. Mullen PE, Pathe M, Purcell R. Stalkers and their victims. New York: Cambridge University Press; 2009.
3. Resnick PJ. Stalking risk assessment. In: Pinals DA, editor. Stalking: psychiatric perspectives and practical approaches. Committee on psychiatry and the law. New York: Oxford University Press; 2007. p. 61–84.
4. Racine C, Billick S. Classification systems for stalking behavior. J Forensic Sci 2014;59(1):250–4.
5. Zona MA, Sharma K, Lane JC. A comparative study of erotomanic and obsessional subjects in a forensic sample. J Forensic Sci 1993;38:894–903.
6. Mohandie K, Meloy JR, McGowan MG, et al. The RECON typology of stalking: reliability and validity based upon a large sample of North American stalkers. J Forensic Sci 2006;51(1):147–55.
7. West SG, Friedman SH. These boots are made for stalking: characteristics of female stalkers. Psychiatry (Edgmont) 2008;5(8):37–42.
8. Meloy JR. Stalking. In: Siegel JA, Saukko PJ, editors. Encyclopedia of forensic sciences. 2nd edition. Waltham (MA): Academic Press; 2013. p. 202–5.
9. Friedman SH. Realistic consideration of women and violence is critical. J Am Acad Psychiatry Law 2015;43(3):273–6.
10. Tjaden P, Thoennes P. Stalking in America: findings from the national violence against women survey. NIJ research in brief U.S. department of justice. Washington, DC: National Institute of Justice; 1998.
11. Purcell R, Pathe M, Mullen PE. A study of women who stalk. Am J Psychiatry 2001;158(12):2056–60.
12. Meloy JR, Boyd C. Female stalkers and their victims. J Am Acad Psychiatry Law 2003;31(2):211–9.
13. Meloy JR, Mohandie K, Green M. The female stalker. Behav Sci Law 2011;29(2): 240–54.
14. Strand S, McEwan TE. Violence among female stalkers. Psychol Med 2012;42(3): 545–55.
15. Evans TM, Meloy JR. Identifying and classifying juvenile stalking behavior. J Forensic Sci 2001;56(Suppl 1):S266–70.

16. Purcell R, Moller B, Flower T, et al. Stalking among juveniles. Br J Psychiatry 2009; 194:451–5.
17. McCann JT. A descriptive study of child and adolescent obsessional followers. J Forensic Sci 2000;45(1):195–9.
18. Purcell R, Pathé M, Mullen PE. Gender differences in stalking behavior among juveniles. J Forens Psychiatry Psychol 2010;21(4):555–68.
19. McIvor RJ, Potter L, Davies L. Stalking behaviour by patients towards psychiatrists in a large mental health organization. Int J Soc Psychiatry 2008;54(4):350–7.
20. Nwachukwu I, Agyapong V, Quinlivan L, et al. Psychiatrists' experiences of stalking in Ireland: prevalence and characteristics. Psychiatrist 2012;36:89–93.
21. Whyte S, Penny C, Christopherson S, et al. The stalking of psychiatrists. Int J Forensic Ment Health 2011;10:254–60.
22. Hughes FA, Thom K, Dixon R. Nature & prevalence of stalking among New Zealand mental health clinicians. J Psychosoc Nurs Ment Health Serv 2007;45(4): 32–9.
23. Sorrentino R, Hatters-Friedman S, Ostermeyer B, et al. An update on stalkers and their victims. Newsl Am Acad Psychiatry Law 2016;41(1):23–7.
24. James DV, Farnham FR. Stalking and serious violence. J Am Acad Psychiatry Law 2003;31(4):432–9.
25. Mastronardi VM, Pomilla A, Ricci S, et al. Stalking of psychiatrists: psychopathological characteristics and gender differences in an Italian sample. Int J Offender Ther Comp Criminol 2013;57(5):526–43.
26. Pathé M, Malloy JR. Commentary: stalking by patients – psychiatrists' tales of anger, lust and ignorance. J Am Acad Psychiatry Law 2013;41:200–5.
27. Dietz P. Assessment of violent threats. Paper Presented at the American Psychiatric Association Annual Meeting, Toronto, May 27-June 4, 1998.
28. Meloy JR. Stalking, an old behavior, a new crime. Psychiatr Clin North Am 1999; 22:85–99.
29. Mechanic MB, Weaver TL, Resick PA. Intimate partner violence and stalking behavior: exploration of patterns and correlates in a sample of acutely battered women. Violence Vict 2000;15:55–72.
30. Zona M, Palarea R, Lane J. Psychiatric diagnosis and the offender victim typology of stalking. In: Meloy JR, editor. The psychology of stalking: clinical and forensic perspectives. San Diego (CA): Academic Press; 1998. p. 69–84.
31. Purcell R, Pathe M, Mullen PE. The prevalence and nature of stalking in the Australian community. Aust N Z J Psychiatry 2002;36:114–20.
32. Purcell R, Pathe M, Mullen PE. When do repeated intrusions become stalking? J Forens Psychiatry Psychol 2004;15:571–83.
33. Rosenfeld B. Recidivism in stalking and obsessional harassment. Law Hum Behav 2003;27(3):251–65.
34. White S, Caywood J. Threat management of stalking cases. In: Meloy JR, editor. The psychology of stalking: clinical and forensic perspectives. San Diego (CA): Academic Press; 1998. p. 98–316.
35. Meloy JR. Stalking and violence. In: Boon J, Sheridan L, editors. Stalking and psychosexual obsession. London: Wiley; 2002. p. 105–24.
36. Resnick PJ. Risk assessment for violence. In: Resnick PJ, editor. Syllabus. Forensic psychiatry review course. Bloomfield (CT): American Academy of Psychiatry and the Law; 2014. p. 105–20.

Sex Offender Risk Assessment and Management

Brad D. Booth, MD, FRCPC[a],*, Drew A. Kingston, PhD[a,b]

KEYWORDS

- Sexual violence • Risk assessment • Risk management
- Mentally disordered offenders

KEY POINTS

- Sexual violence is common and requires an organized approach for risk assessment and risk management. Current evidence-based risk assessment should include actuarial and structured professional judgment tools.
- Mental illness in sexual offenders is also frequent. Although evidence does not suggest that it usually contributes to recidivism, it can influence treatment of sexual offending in this population. Risk management should include treatment of comorbid psychiatric conditions.
- Risk management strategies for sexual violence include external control measures, psychotherapeutic approaches, and pharmacologic approaches. However, quality research proving the efficacy of these interventions is lacking and further research is needed.
- Despite limited data, risk management strategies should combine cognitive-behavioral interventions designed to target criminogenic factors based on Risk-Need-Responsivity principles, but Good Lives interventions may also help.
- Pharmacologic interventions should include consideration of selective serotonin reuptake inhibitors and antitestosterone agents, depending on the analysis of risk.

INTRODUCTION

Of all forms of violence, sexual violence can cause the most profound effects on victims. Sexual violence includes forced sexual contact on a spectrum from unwelcome touching to penetration. It can escalate to physical violence and sadistic behaviors by the perpetrator. It also includes sexual contact with those who cannot ethically

Disclosure: The authors have nothing to disclose.
[a] Integrated Forensic Program, Royal Ottawa Mental Health Care Group, Department of Psychiatry, University of Ottawa, 1145 Carling Avenue, Ottawa, Ontario K1Z 7K4, Canada; [b] Brockville Mental Health Centre (BMHC), 1804 Highway 2 East, PO Box 1050, Brockville, Ontario K6V 5W7, Canada
* Corresponding author. 2nd Floor – Forensics, 1145 Carling Avenue, Ottawa, Ontario K1Z 7K4, Canada.
E-mail address: brad.booth@theroyal.ca

Psychiatr Clin N Am 39 (2016) 675–689
http://dx.doi.org/10.1016/j.psc.2016.07.011
0193-953X/16/© 2016 Elsevier Inc. All rights reserved.

psych.theclinics.com

consent, such as children or intellectually disabled individuals. Usually noncontact sexual offending, such as child pornography possession or voyeurism, is not considered sexual violence. Although the rates of sexual violence have been decreasing since the early 1990s, this decrease seems to mainly be in lower level offenses with the least injury to the victim.[1,2] Rates of sexual assault remain unacceptably high with approximately 19% of women and 1.7% of men in the United States reporting they have been sexually assaulted during their lifetimes.[3] Similarly, rates of childhood sexual abuse range from 7% to 36% for women and from 3% to 29% for men.[4]

The emotional toll for victims of sexual violence is profound.[1] Many victims experience fear and anger. Many do not report the assault to police and may not disclose the violence to anyone. Victims can be left with permanent psychiatric disability, including depression, posttraumatic stress disorder (PTSD), and other sequelae.

Given these issues, appropriate risk assessment and risk management of sexual violence is paramount. This article outlines the evidence-based approach to assist clinicians working with this type of violence.

RISK ASSESSMENT OF SEXUAL VIOLENCE
Evaluation Stage

The first step of comprehensive risk assessment of sexual violence is a comprehensive evaluation, described previously.[5] This includes:

- Familiarizing yourself with the relevant legislation (eg, specific wording of sexually violent predator law) and clarify the medicolegal questions you are addressing.
- Reviewing collateral information, including details of any current and previous offenses, institutional records, transcripts from court proceedings, mental health and treatment records, school records, and other information that might be available.
- Completing a clinical interview of the offender focusing on details of sexual offending, risk factors, and any treatable psychiatric comorbidities.
- Performing sexual preference testing if available, such as phallometric testing[6,7] or Abel testing.[8]
- Performing adjunctive tests as appropriate (eg, IQ [intelligence quotient] testing, attention-deficit/hyperactivity disorder [ADHD] testing, neuropsychological profile, malingering, personality testing).

Usually this assessment only occurs after a finding of guilt to avoid undue influence on the fact finder. Once a comprehensive evaluation has taken place, then the risk assessment is based on the specific issues raised by the offending and case-specific issues of the offender. Although rates of sexual offending recidivism are approximately 13% for all untreated sexual offenders,[9,10] the risk of a particular offender could be much higher or lower depending on the offender's history.

Structured Risk Assessment

Risk assessment of sexual offenders has become increasingly important to criminal justice decision making. Only professionals trained and experienced in the assessment and treatment of this population should perform risk assessment of this nature. Professionals may choose from various methods to assess the risk for violence.[11] Historically, unstructured professional judgment was the norm, such that clinicians based their decisions on personal experience. However, this approach has shown poor predictive accuracy.[12–14]

Current approaches are usually divided into actuarial measures and structured professional judgment. Most validated measures are actuarial. These measures contain a fixed number of items with specified decision-making rules for scoring. Items contained in these scales are typically based on research showing an empirical link to recidivism[15] and these items combine to provide probabilistic estimates of the likelihood of a new offense. Applied on a large scale, actuarial methods seem to have the highest accuracy in predicting recidivism.[12,16] However, actuarial measures have been criticized as mathematically flawed when applied to individual offenders for the risk the person may pose.[17]

Structured professional judgment tools involve organized evaluation of risk factors that are empirically related to recidivism along with items that are considered to be clinically important. Risk assessors make judgments about risk to reoffend after considering the list of factors, without probabilistic estimates. These tools have also been shown to have good validity in the assessment of risk.[12,18]

A detailed review of all actuarial risk assessment measures and structured professional guides is beyond the scope of this article. Some of the more common risk assessment tools in the past have included the Static-99,[19] the Static-2002,[20] the Violence Risk Appraisal Guide (VRAG) and the Sex Offender Risk Appraisal Guide (SORAG),[21] the Sex Offender Screening Tool (SOST),[22] and the Sexual Violence Risk-20 (SVR-20).[23] Some of these measures are predominantly composed of static (ie, historical) risk factors such as criminal history. However, dynamic risk factors, such as presence of social supports, have also been shown to be important to assess change in risk. These dynamic factors help to provide a framework of understanding of the individual, which can assist in developing intervention strategies to reduce recidivism. As such, the analysis of dynamic risk factors has been incorporated into some tools. The Stable-2007 and Acute-2007 are measures that differentiate between stable and acute dynamic risk factors and have been shown to be predictive of recidivism.[24]

However, although the original scales noted earlier were initially shown as having fair validity, further research showed these instruments to have various flaws. As such, many tools have been revised and improved. The current iterations of these tools are the Static-99R and the Static-2002R (which correct for age),[25] the Violence Risk Appraisal Guide - Revised (VRAG-R) (which replaces both the VRAG and SORAG),[26] and the Minnesota Sex Offender Screening Tool - 3.1 (Mn-SOST-3.1) (which replaces the Sex Offender Screening Tool (SOST) and the Minnesota Sex Offender Screening Tool (Mn-SOST).[27] Further, actuarial risk tables citing rates of recidivism in these tools have also been adjusted variable numbers of times. These revisions highlight that, although effective in assisting to assess risk, the tools are limited by the science available and no tool is 100% accurate.

Given the variety of risk appraisal tools available, it can be difficult for clinicians to select the most appropriate one to assess risk for recidivism. Although the use of multiple measures in risk assessment is common, interpretation becomes difficult when divergent measures produce discrepant findings (see Barbaree and colleagues[28]). In addition, research pertaining to the added value of multiple measures is mixed. For example, Seto[29] found that the combination of multiple risk measures did not improve predictive accuracy in risk assessment with sexual offenders. Some more recent studies have shown that use of multiple actuarial instruments can add incrementally to the prediction of recidivism.[30]

Clinical Factors in Risk Assessment

Although actuarial and structured professional judgment tools attempt to standardize and simplify risk assessment, Hanson and colleagues[31] noted that these tools are not meant to be used alone and that factors outside of the tools may also be important. Individuals when evaluated may have important issues for risk that are not accounted for in actuarial or structured professional judgment tools. For example, if an offender becomes quadriplegic, the risk may decrease exponentially but this would not be accounted for in most standardized assessment tools. Similarly, an offender may develop a psychotic delusion that they must commit a sexual offense. Alternatively, one factor for an individual may be extremely important (eg, history of sexual homicide), but not given weight in standard assessment tools. As such, a combination of actuarial methods and structured professional judgment combined with clinical adjustments to risk assessment based on the clinical assessment of the offender is recommended.

Part of the clinical analysis of risk for individual offenders uses the evaluation of specific factors relevant to that particular offender. For high-stakes assessments, this should include an assessment of psychopathy using a validated scale such as the Hare Psychopathy Checklist (PCL-R).[32] Although only a single risk factor among many, presence of psychopathy suggests decreased treatability and increased risk.[33–36]

Offenders should also be evaluated for the presence of paraphilic disorders[37] and hypersexual disorders.[38] Among child molesters, the presence of pedophilic disorder has been shown to increase risk of recidivism.[9] However, some investigators have questioned the utility of phallometric testing and a pedophilia diagnosis.[39–42] Hypersexual disorders and sexual preoccupation may also be relevant factors.[10,15,43–45]

Psychiatrists and psychologists also bring specialized skill in diagnosing mental disorders, which may be present and relevant in particular sexual offenders. The relationship between mental illness and offending is complex. Some investigators think that mental illness increases the risk of recidivism in some individuals.[46–48] Large-scale studies suggest that mental illness is not usually a criminogenic factor related to recidivism.[49–53] Although presence of mental illness does not seem to predict recidivism in most individuals, it may interfere with responsiveness to treatment of sexual offending. It may also be relevant in assessing the offending of individual offenders.

Separate from this controversy, most investigators accept that the rate of mental illness among prisoners is high.[54–56] Although mental illness rates among general offenders have been studied, rates of mental illness among sexual offenders are less known. Limited studies suggest increased rates of mood disorders, psychosis, anxiety disorders, substance use disorders, ADHD, neurocognitive disorders, and intellectual/developmental disorders.[57–61] Within our facility for offenders with mental illness serving jail sentences, rates of mental illness among sexual offenders were 43% for depressive disorders, 13% for bipolar disorder, 28% for anxiety disorders, 16% for psychotic disorders, 10% for dementia, 31% for mental retardation/developmental delay, 42% for alcohol dependence, 38% for substance dependence, 20% for ADHD, and 47% for personality disorders.[62] A more recent study of sexual offenders more than 55 years old yielded a rate of 62% (26 of 42) of the sample with neurocognitive disorders.[63] The index of suspicion for these disorders should be high and all offenders should be evaluated for psychiatric illness. These disorders may have relevance to the offender's particular risk assessment and risk management.

RISK MANAGEMENT OF SEXUAL VIOLENCE

Once the risk of sexual violence has been evaluated, the next step is to evaluate how to manage that risk for that particular offender. Management strategies should be tailored to the offender's risk, needs, and the availability of resources. Although there may be societal pressure for harsh sentencing as the only risk management strategy, this narrow approach is financially prohibitive[64] and does not address the risk management needs of offenders once they are reintegrated into society. Strict sentencing may have a valid basis in justice principles and the need to punish, but should not be confused with risk management. In reality, most sexual offenders do not recidivate and even very-high-risk individuals can be successfully managed in the community.[65] Ideally, risk management strategies balance the actual (not perceived) risk that the individual poses with the limited community resources, with fiscal responsibility and with the liberty interests of the offender. The least-restrictive and least-onerous strategies that are scientifically validated should be used. Risk management strategies can be broken down into:

- External control
- Psychotherapy-based treatments
- Pharmacotherapy treatments
- Treatment of comorbidities

External Control

The external control mechanisms for sexual offenders are generally based in the legal system. These mechanisms can include strict sentencing and mandatory minimum sentences. In Canada, the Criminal Code allows for indeterminate sentencing of dangerous offenders to manage risk (not to punish). Thus, a violent offender or sexual offender can be incarcerated indefinitely, until such time as the offender can show the parole board that the risk posed by placement in the community can be safely managed. For some, this may mean never entering the community.

In the United States, similar mechanisms exist in the form of sexually violent predator laws (eg, see Booth and Schmedlen[66]), which are civil commitment laws generally given at the end of a sentence based on the fact that the individual has a legally defined mental disorder and poses a risk. These strategies have some rationale, because there are offenders who will remain too high risk to be managed in the community. In addition, it is generally recognized that risk of sexual recidivism decreases with age so that longer incarceration allows for a natural desistence from offending.[67–69] This approach can be prohibitively expensive, taking public monies away from other societal needs.

When a sexual offender does enter the community, probation or parole officers often monitor and support the offender. To supplement this, one approach to control risk is requiring signing on to sex offender registries or notifying the public about offenders entering the community. Although likely providing some reassurance to the public and potentially serving as a resource for police, the utility in decreasing recidivism has been questioned.[70,71] Another strategy uses zoning restrictions (eg, not living within a certain distance from schools) or requiring offenders to have global positioning system (GPS) tracking. Again, these strategies have not been shown to be helpful and may increase risk of homelessness, making tracking and providing risk-reducing interventions difficult.[72]

Psychotherapy-based Interventions

Treatment of sexual offending behavior should be multipronged. Psychotherapy-based interventions currently focus on cognitive-behavioral models of therapy. The current treatment of choice for sexual offenders adheres to the principles of effective correctional intervention,[73] in which treatment is matched to the risk posed by individual offenders (risk principle), specifically targets criminogenic needs (need principle), and is tailored to the individual learning styles and abilities of offenders (responsivity principle). The Risk-Need-Responsivity (RNR) Model of treatment of sexual offenders stems from the General Personality and Cognitive Social Learning theory.[73] The theory suggests that there are 8 risk factors (ie, The Big 8) supported in the literature that are linked to recidivism:

- Criminal history
- Procriminal companions
- Procriminal attitudes
- Antisocial personality pattern
- Education/employment
- Family/marital factors
- Substance abuse
- Leisure/recreation

Thus, treatment programs should include cognitive-behavioral interventions and be aimed at these targets. This approach has a large research basis supporting efficacy.[74,75]

An alternative approach, coined the Good Lives Model,[76] is also seen in sex offender treatment programs. This program is strengths based, which helps offenders gain internal and external resources to live a good or better life; a life that is socially acceptable and personally meaningful. Briefly, according to the principles of the Good Lives Model, treatment should proceed on the assumption that effective reha-bilitation requires the acquisition of competencies and external supports necessary to achieve a better Good Lives plan. Thus, the goal of treatment is to enhance human well-being (ie, Good Lives), with the expectation that this will aid in reducing risk by assisting individuals to acquire particular goods and to achieve goals in prosocial, nonoffending ways. Consequently, the offender will be able to achieve a satisfying, ful-filling life that is incompatible with sexual offending. Compared with RNR, the Good Lives Model has been subject to much more limited empirical support.[77]

Despite major resource investment in therapies, the research literature remains lacking to support these therapies. This lack is in part caused by the low base rate of recidivism among sexual offenders, with about 13% reoffending in 5 years.[9,15] Thus, even programs providing large services have few individuals reoffend. Several meta-analyses have suggested that cognitive-behavioral treatment strategies are effective in reducing recidivism.[78–82] Other large-scale studies have suggested limited effectiveness, particularly for the relapse-prevention approach.[83–85] Much of the diffi-culty comes from research methodologies and low base rates resulting in a recom-mendation for further study.[86–88] With these caveats, psychological treatment is recommended.

Pharmacotherapy Interventions

Although psychological treatment is always encouraged, pharmacologic interventions to mitigate the risk of sexual violence should always be considered. Treatment targets broadly include endocrine targets to reduce testosterone levels and neurotransmitter targets such as serotonin,[89] both with a goal of reducing sexual drive. Detailed analyses of the mechanism of action of various agents, treatment algorithms, and ef-ficacy of these medications are available in the literature.[86,90–95] As with psychological interventions, the evidence for recommending treatments is limited, again because of low base rates of recidivism and difficulties developing acceptable research designs. As a result, all medications are currently off label and should be used with caution.

With this caveat, there is some evidence to recommend the use of selective seroto-nin reuptake inhibitors (SSRIs). The mechanism of action may be by inhibition of sexual activity through serotonin's direct effect on reducing libido. Serotonergic medications may also reduce impulsiveness and have an effect on the obsessive-compulsive na-ture of paraphilias. There may also be indirect effects on testosterone levels. Options include sertraline 50 mg to 150 mg daily, paroxetine 10 mg to 30 mg daily, citalopram 20 mg to 40 mg daily, or other serotonergic agents.

When SSRIs are ineffective or the risk of the offender too high, then hormonal treat-ments are recommended. These medications all have the effect of reducing free testosterone level. Leydig cells in the testes produce testosterone in response to stim-ulation by luteinizing hormone (LH) released by the anterior pituitary gland. LH release is controlled by the pulsatile release of gonadotropin-releasing hormone (GNRH) from the hypothalamus. Medications affecting this pathway can include those that directly block testosterone at a cellular level, such as cyproterone acetate at oral doses of 50 mg to 400 mg daily (not available in the United States). Alternatively, negative feed-back mechanisms can be used, such as giving medroxyprogesterone, which results in a reduction in LH level and subsequent reduced testosterone production in the testes. Doses in sexual offenders are typically 100 mg to 600 mg orally per day or 100 mg to 700 mg intramuscularly every week or two. In addition, GNRH agonists can be given by injection to produce a high steady state of GNRH, with a subsequent decrease of LH and testosterone levels to near-castrate levels. Options include leuprolide (7.5 mg monthly or 22.5 mg every 3 months), goserelin (3.6 mg monthly or 10.8 mg every 3 months), or triptorelin (3.75 mg per month or 11.25 mg every 3 months). The benefits of these interventions must be weighed against the risks and they should be only given if medically safe with appropriate medical consultation and monitoring.

Choosing the appropriate agent should include an evaluation of risk (likelihood and severity) in addition to monitoring requirements, patient reliability, health of the patient, patient preference, and availability of these agents. There have been several algo-rithms developed outlining different approaches.[86,90,91] In general, the least intrusive and restrictive measure should be sought that is appropriate to the individual.

Treatment of Comorbidities

As noted earlier, the role of mental illness as a risk factor for criminal recidivism is un-clear. However, most evidence suggests that it is not criminogenic on a large scale. Presence of mental illness may even be protective for some individuals. However, illness can interfere with provision of a Risk-Need-Responsivity–based treatment pro-gram. Some individuals may become an acute risk when ill; for example, if psychotic and disinhibited. Further, treatment providers who do not work with mentally ill of-fenders may not recognize illness and may assume that the offender is not interested in treatment or is intentionally disruptive. However, there are no validated studies to suggest the best approach in treating mentally disordered sexual offenders and clinical experience provides most guidance.

Mood disorders

Depression and bipolar illness are seen in some sexual offenders. The process of arrest, legal hearings, and incarceration often results in numerous losses, including family supports, finances, and social status. Thus, depression is expected. Depressive episodes can cause apathy, low motivation, concentration problems, hopelessness, suicidality, and psychomotor slowing or agitation. In more severe episodes, some in-dividuals also get psychotic symptoms. Depressive symptoms can interfere with cognitive-behavioral sex offender treatment because participation and homework completion can be compromised. Offenders may require pharmacologic treatment, therapy, or even electroconvulsive therapy to improve their depression before entering a group. SSRIs could have the benefit of helping with depression and decreasing sexual drive. Although depression can interfere with treatment, entering a supportive group milieu may have some benefits on the depression.

Manic or hypomanic episodes can also be induced by psychosocial stressors of the trial or of incarceration. Both of these states cause great difficulty in effectively participating in groups and are likely to be a relative contraindication to entering sex offender therapy.

Anxiety disorders

The broad range of anxiety disorders can also be relevant to sexual offender treatment. Individuals with social anxiety disorder have difficulties attending and participating in group therapy. Further, the associated fear of social judgment may contribute to seeking out younger/less-intimidating social outlets (eg, children), thus contributing to offending. Individuals with sexual offenses are also at higher risk of themselves having been abused,[96] which could result in PTSD. These offenders may have flashbacks and other PTSD symptoms from groups focused on detailed accounts of offenses. Further, these individuals often are not welcome in treatment groups for those who have childhood abuse. Panic disorder, obsessive-compulsive disorder, and generalized anxiety disorder may also be relevant, although they tend to interfere less in general sex offender treatment. Again, treatment with SSRIs may serve dual benefits for treatment of anxiety and sexual drive.

Psychotic disorders

Most offender treatment programs are not equipped to deal with seriously mentally ill individuals, particularly those with psychotic disorders. Active psychosis causes impaired reality testing, disorganized thinking, hallucinations, and delusions. These symptoms could be disruptive to group process. Further, many individuals with psychotic illness have negative symptoms of illness with paucity of thought, paucity of speech, amotivation, and other symptoms. These symptoms also pose difficulty in most treatment groups. Active psychosis is a relative contraindication to sex offender treatment and should usually be stabilized first. These individuals often need specialized supports for reintegration into the community.

Neurocognitive disorders

Neurocognitive disorders, such as dementia, seem to be increasingly relevant in offender populations and pose particular challenges in the correctional setting.[63,97–99] Dementia may go unrecognized and clinicians should screen offenders who are more than 50 years old. Memory issues and other problems of aging (hearing deficits, sight deficits, physical mobility issues) can interfere with benefits in groups. Although older age seems to decrease risk of recidivism,[100,101] dementia likely can disinhibit some offenders and may be linked in some individuals to offending. Discharge planning can also be complicated by increased health care needs, stigma, and lack of support.

Attention-deficit/hyperactivity disorder

ADHD is present at increased rates among general offenders and in some studies in sexual offenders.[58,102,103] Symptoms include attention difficulties. Untreated, this could interfere with listening in groups, staying focused, consolidation of learning, and completing assignments. Further, impulsivity issues may interfere with appropriate group dynamics and may be relevant to offending. Treatment of ADHD may be needed, although concerns about medication diversion and abuse need to be considered. In addition to better functioning in groups, treatment of ADHD has been shown to reduce criminality.[104] Limited data suggest that stimulant medications for ADHD may even decrease paraphilic interest in some individuals.[105]

SUMMARY

Sexual violence is common. When faced with individuals who perpetrate sexual violence, an organized approach for evaluation is required. Clarification of diagnosis and understanding of the individual is paramount. A scientifically validated risk assessment is required, combining actuarial measures with structured professional judgment tools to refine the understanding of risk for that individual. Clinical experience and expertise assist in this regard and can provide important adjustments to risk evaluation.

Once the individual's risk for recurrent sexual violence is clarified, thought is required to design a risk management plan that balances the risk the individual poses with the costs, available resources, and needs of the offender. Treatment programs are typically based on principles underscored by either the Risk-Need-Responsivity Model or the Good Lives Model. Although the efficacy of psychotherapy-based interventions for sexual offenders continues to be debated with emphasis placed on the method in which such program are evaluated,[106,107] the evidence suggests that treatment can have a positive effect on the individual's risk of recidivism.[81] Clinicians therefore should use current best practices in offender rehabilitation and appropriately customize these approaches to the specific needs of the offender. Clarification and treatment of psychiatric comorbidity can help to shape these services. Ultimately, these interventions will serve to reduce sexual violence in the future.

REFERENCES

1. Brennan S, Taylor-Butts A. Canadian Centre for Justice statistics profile series. Sexual assault in Canada: 2004 and 2007. Ottawa (Canada): Ministry of Industry; 2008.
2. Planty M, Langton L. Special report: female victims of sexual violence, 1994-2010. Bureau of Justice Statistics; 2013.
3. Breiding MJ, Smith SG, Basile KC, et al. Prevalence and characteristics of sexual violence, stalking, and intimate partner violence victimization–national intimate partner and sexual violence survey, United States, 2011. MMWR Surveill Summ 2014;63(8):1–18.
4. Finkelhor D. The international epidemiology of child sexual abuse. Child Abuse Negl 1994;18(5):409–17.
5. Bradford JM, Seto MC, Booth BD. Forensic assessment of sex offenders. In: Simon RI, Gold LH, editors. The American Psychiatric Publishing textbook of forensic psychiatry. 2nd edition. Washington, DC: American Psychiatric Association Press; 2010. p. 373–94.
6. Zuckerman M. Physiological measures of sexual arousal in the human. Psychol Bull 1971;75(5):297–329.
7. Bancroft JH, Jones HG, Pullan BR. A simple transducer for measuring penile erection with comments on its use in the treatment of sexual disorders. Behav Res Ther 1966;4(3):239–41.
8. Abel GG, Huffman J, Warberg B, et al. Visual reaction time and plethysmography as measures of sexual interest in child molesters. Sex Abuse 1998; 10(2):81–95.

9. Hanson RK, Bussiere MT. Predicting relapse: a meta-analysis of sexual offender recidivism studies. J Consult Clin Psychol 1998;66(2):348–62.

10. Hanson RK, Morton-Bourgon KE. Predictors of sexual recidivism: an updated meta-analysis. Ottawa (Canada): Public Safety and Emergency Preparedness Canada; 2004.

11. Douglas KS, Hart SD, Webster CD, et al. HCR-20 (Version 3): assessing risk for violence. Burnaby (Canada): Mental Health, Law, and Policy Institute, Simon Fraser University; 2013.

12. Hanson RK, Morton-Bourgon KE. The accuracy of recidivism risk assessments for sexual offenders: a meta-analysis of 118 prediction studies. Psychol Assess 2009;21(1):1–21.

13. Hanson RK, Morton KE, Harris AJ. Sexual offender recidivism risk: what we know and what we need to know. Ann N Y Acad Sci 2003;989:154–66 [discussion: 236–46].

14. Hanson RK. Twenty years of progress in violence risk assessment. J Interpers Violence 2005;20(2):212–7.

15. Hanson RK, Morton-Bourgon KE. The characteristics of persistent sexual offenders: a meta-analysis of recidivism studies. J Consult Clin Psychol 2005; 73(6):1154–63.

16. Grove WM, Zald DH, Lebow BS, et al. Clinical versus mechanical prediction: a meta-analysis. Psychol Assess 2000;12(1):19–30.

17. Hart SD, Michie C, Cooke DJ. Precision of actuarial risk assessment instruments: evaluating the 'margins of error' of group v. individual predictions of violence. Br J Psychiatry Suppl 2007;190(49):s60–5.

18. de Vogel V, de Ruiter C, van Beek D, et al. Predictive validity of the SVR-20 and Static-99 in a Dutch sample of treated sex offenders. Law Hum Behav 2004; 28(3):235–51.

19. Hanson RK, Thornton D. Improving risk assessments for sex offenders: a comparison of three actuarial scales. Law Hum Behav 2000;24(1):119–36.

20. Hanson RK, Thornton D. Corrections research user report no. 2003-01. Notes on the development of the Static-2002. Ottawa (Canada): Department of the Solicitor General of Canada; 2003.

21. Quinsey VL, Harris GT, Rice ME, et al. Violent offenders: appraising and managing risk. 2nd edition. Washington, DC: American Psychological Association; 2006.

22. Epperson DL, Kaul JD, Huot SJ. Predicting the risk for recidivism for incarcerated sex offenders: updated development on the Sex Offender Screening Tool (SOST). Annual Conference of the Association for the Treatment of Sexual Abusers. New Orleans (LA), October 1995.

23. Boer DP, Hart SD, Kropp PR, et al. Manual for the sexual violence risk-20. Professional guidelines for assessing risk of sexual violence. Vancouver (Canada): Institute Against Family Violence; 1997.

24. Hanson RK, Harris AJR, Scott T-L, et al. Assessing the risk of sexual offender on community supervision: the Dynamic Supervision Project. Corrections research user report 2007-05. Ottawa (Canada): Public Safety Canada; 2007.

25. Helmus L, Thornton D, Hanson RK, et al. Improving the predictive accuracy of Static-99 and Static-2002 with older sex offenders: revised age weights. Sex Abuse 2012;24(1):64–101.

26. Rice ME, Harris GT, Lang C. Validation of and revision to the VRAG and SORAG: the Violence Risk Appraisal Guide-Revised (VRAG-R). Psychol Assess 2013; 25(3):951–65.

27. Duwe G, Freske P. The Minnesota Sex Offender Screening Tool-3.1 (MnSOST-3.1). In: Phenix A, Hoberman MH, editors. Sexual offending: predisposing antecedents, assessments and management. New York: Springer; 2016. p. 489–502.

28. Barbaree HE, Langton CM, Peacock EJ. Different actuarial risk measures produce different risk rankings for sexual offenders. Sex Abuse 2006;18(4):423–40.

29. Seto MC. Is more better? Combining actuarial risk scales to predict recidivism among adult sex offenders. Psychol Assess 2005;17(2):156–67.

30. Babchishin KM, Hanson RK, Helmus L. Even highly correlated measures can add incrementally to predicting recidivism among sex offenders. Assessment 2012;19(4):442–61.

31. Hanson RK, Thornton D, Helmus LM, et al. What sexual recidivism rates are associated with Static-99R and Static-2002R scores? Sex Abuse 2016;28(3): 218–52.

32. Hare R. Hare psychopathy checklist revised (PCL-R). 2nd edition. Toronto: Multi-Health Systems; 2003.

33. Kingston DA, Firestone P, Wexler A, et al. Factors associated with recidivism among intrafamilial child molesters. J Sex Aggress 2008;14(1):3–18.

34. Langton CM, Barbaree HE, Harkins L, et al. Sex offenders' response to treatment and its association with recidivism as a function of psychopathy. Sex Abuse 2006;18(1):99–120.

35. Barbaree HE. Psychopathy, treatment behavior, and recidivism: an extended follow-up of Seto and Barbaree. J Interpers Violence 2005;20(9):1115–31.

36. Harris AJR. The psychopathy checklist, screening version: applications with parole and probation sex offender samples. Ottawa, Canada: Carleton University; 2003.

37. American Psychiatric Association. Diagnostic and statistical manual of mental disorders. 5th edition. Arlington (VA): American Psychiatric Publishing; 2013.

38. Kafka MP. Hypersexual disorder: a proposed diagnosis for DSM-V. Arch Sex Behav 2010;39(2):377–400.

39. Kingston DA, Firestone P, Moulden HM, et al. The utility of the diagnosis of pedophilia: a comparison of various classification procedures. Arch Sex Behav 2007; 36(3):423–36.

40. Marshall WL. Clinical and research limitations in the use of phallometric testing with sexual offenders. Sex Offender Treat 2006;1(1):1–19.

41. Marshall WL. Diagnostic problems with sexual offenders. In: Marshall WL, Fernandez YM, Marshall LE, et al, editors. Sexual offender treatment: controversial issues. New York: John Wiley; 2006. p. 33–43.

42. Marshall WL, Fernandez YM. Phallometric testing with sexual offenders: limits to its value. Clin Psychol Rev 2000;20(7):807–22.

43. Marshall L, Marshall W. Sexual addiction in incarcerated sexual offenders. Sex Addict Compul 2006;13(4):377–90.

44. Kafka MP. Sex offending and sexual appetite: the clinical and theoretical relevance of hypersexual desire. Int J Offender Ther Comp Criminol 2003;47(4): 439–51.

45. Kingston DA, Bradford JM. Hypersexuality and recidivism among sexual offenders. Sex Addict Compul 2013;20(1–2):91–105.

46. Craig LA, Giotakos O. Sexual offending in psychotic patients. In: Boer DP, Eher R, Craig LA, et al, editors. International perspectives on the assessment and treatment of sexual offenders: theory, practice, and research. Chichester, West Sussex: Wiley-Blackwell; 2011. p. 463–78.

47. Stinson JD, Becker JV. Sexual offenders with serious mental illness: prevention, risk, and clinical concerns. Int J Law Psychiatry 2011;34(3):239–45.

48. Langstrom N, Sjostedt G, Grann M. Psychiatric disorders and recidivism in sexual offenders. Sex Abuse 2004;16(2):139–50.

49. Bonta J, Blais B, Wilson HA. The prediction of risk for mentally disordered offenders: a quantitative synthesis. User report 2013-01. Ottawa (Canada): Public Safety Canada; 2013.

50. Phillips HK, Gray NS, MacCulloch SI, et al. Risk assessment in offenders with mental disorders: relative efficacy of personal demographic, criminal history, and clinical variables. J Interpers Violence 2005;20(7):833–47.

51. Bonta J, Law M, Hanson K. The prediction of criminal and violent recidivism among mentally disordered offenders: a meta-analysis. Psychol Bull 1998; 123(2):123–42.

52. Kingston DA, Olver ME, Harris M, et al. The relationship between mental illness and violence in a mentally disordered offender sample: evaluating criminogenic and psychopathological predictors. Psychol Crime Law 2016;22:678–700.

53. Kingston DA, Olver ME, Harris M, et al. The relationship between mental disorder and recidivism in sexual offenders. Int J Forensic Ment Health 2015;14(1): 10–22.

54. Torrey EF, Kennard AD, Eslinger D, et al. More mentally ill persons are in jails and prisons than hospitals: a survey of the states. Alexandria (VA): National Sheriffs Association; 2010.

55. Harcourt BE. From the asylum to the prison: rethinking the incarceration revolution. Tex Law Rev 2006;84(7):1751–86.

56. Konrad N. Prisons as new asylums. Curr Opin Psychiatry 2002;15(6):583–7.

57. Dunsieth NW Jr, Nelson EB, Brusman-Lovins LA, et al. Psychiatric and legal features of 113 men convicted of sexual offenses. J Clin Psychiatry 2004;65(3): 293–300.

58. Kafka MP, Hennen J. A DSM-IV Axis I comorbidity study of males (n = 120) with paraphilias and paraphilia-related disorders. Sex Abuse 2002;14(4):349–66.

59. Kafka MP, Prentky RA. Preliminary observations of DSM-III-R Axis I comorbidity in men with paraphilias and paraphilia-related disorders. J Clin Psychiatry 1994; 55(11):481–7.

60. McElroy SL, Soutullo CA, Taylor P Jr, et al. Psychiatric features of 36 men convicted of sexual offenses. J Clin Psychiatry 1999;60(6):414–20 [quiz: 421–2].

61. Raymond NC, Coleman E, Ohlerking F, et al. Psychiatric comorbidity in pedophilic sex offenders. Am J Psychiatry 1999;156(5):786–8.

62. Booth BD. Special populations: mentally disordered sexual offenders (MDSOs). In: Harrison K, editor. Managing high-risk sex offenders in the community: risk management, treatment and social responsibilities. Devon: Willan Publishing; 2010.

63. Booth BD, Ranger RC, Harris M, et al. Elderly sexual offenders – prevalence and management issues. Paper presented at Annual Meeting of the American Academy of Psychiatry and the Law. Fort Lauderdale (FL), October 2015.

64. La Fond JQ. The costs of enacting a sexual predator law. Psychology, Public Policy, and the Law 1998;4(1):468–504.

65. Harrison K. Managing high-risk sex offenders in the community: risk management, treatment and social responsibilities. Devon: Willan Publishing; 2010.

66. Booth BD, Schmedlen G. Sexually violent predators laws. J Am Acad Psychiatry Law 2006;34(4):553–5.

67. Nicholaichuk TP, Olver ME, Gu D, et al. Age, actuarial risk and long-term recidivism in a national sample of sex offenders. Sex Abuse 2014;26(5):406–28.

68. Hanson RK, Harris AJ, Helmus L, et al. High-risk sex offenders may not be high risk forever. J Interpers Violence 2014;29(15):2792–813.

69. Wollert R, Cramer E, Waggoner J, et al. Recent research (N = 9,305) underscores the importance of using age-stratified actuarial tables in sex offender risk assessments. Sex Abuse 2010;22(4):471–90.

70. Prescott JJ, Rockoff JE. Do sex offender registration and notification laws affect criminal behavior? J Law Econ 2011;54(1):161–206.

71. Agan AY. Sex offender registries: fear without function? J Law Econ 2011;54(1): 207–39.

72. Barton RA, Wesley RW, Spillane SR. Special review: assessment of electronic monitoring of sex offenders on parole and the impact of residency restrictions. California; 2014. Available at: http://www.oig.ca.gov/media/reports/Reports/Reviews/OIG_Special_Review_Electronic_Monitoring_of_Sex_Offenders_on_Parole_and_Impact_of_Residency_Restrictions_November_2014.pdf. Accessed June 30, 2016.

73. Andrews DA, Bonta J. The psychology of criminal conduct. 5th edition. New Providence (NJ): Matthew Bender & Company; 2010.

74. Hanson RK, Bourgon G, Helmus L, et al. A meta-analysis of the effectiveness of treatment for sexual offenders: risk, need, and responsivity. Ottawa (Canada): Public Safety Canada; 2009.

75. Hanson RK, Morton-Bourgon KE. The accuracy of recidivism risk assessments for sexual offenders: a meta-analysis. Ottawa (Canada): Public Safety and Emergency Preparedness Canada; 2007.

76. Ward T, Yates PM, Willis GM. The Good Lives Model and the Risk Need Responsivity Model: a critical response to Andrews, Bonta, and Wormith (2011). Crim Justice Behav 2012;39(1):94–110.

77. Marshall LE, Marshall WL, Fernandez YM, et al. The Rockwood Preparatory Program for sexual offenders: description and preliminary appraisal. Sex Abuse 2008;20(1):25–42.

78. Alexander MA. Sexual offender treatment efficacy revisited. Sex Abuse 1999; 11(2):101–16.

79. Hall GC. Sexual offender recidivism revisited: a meta-analysis of recent treatment studies. J Consult Clin Psychol 1995;63(5):802–9.

80. Gallagher C, Wilson DB, Hirshfield P, et al. A quantitative review of the effects of sex offender treatment on sexual reoffending. Correct Manag Q 1999;3:19–29.

81. Hanson RK, Gordon A, Harris AJ, et al. First report of the collaborative outcome data project on the effectiveness of psychological treatment for sex offenders. Sex Abuse 2002;14(2):169–94 [discussion: 195–7].

82. Lösel F, Schmucker M. The effectiveness of treatment for sexual offenders: a comprehensive meta-analysis. J Exp Criminol 2005;1(1):117–46.

83. Marques JK, Wiederanders M, Day DM, et al. Effects of a relapse prevention program on sexual recidivism: final results from California's Sex Offender Treatment and Evaluation Project (SOTEP). Sex Abuse 2005;17(1):79–107.

84. Furby L, Weinrott MR, Blackshaw L. Sex offender recidivism: a review. Psychol Bull 1989;105(1):3–30.

85. Grønnerød C, Grønnerød JS, Grøndahl P. Psychological treatment of sexual offenders against children: a meta-analytic review of treatment outcome studies. Trauma Violence Abuse 2015;16(3):280–90.

86. Thibaut F, de la Barra F, Gordon H, et al. The World Federation of Societies of Biological Psychiatry (WFSBP) guidelines for the biological treatment of paraphilias. World J Biol Psychiatr 2010;11:604–55.

87. Hanson RK. Review: evidence does not support a reduction in sexual reoffending with psychological interventions, but further high-quality trials are needed. Evid Based Ment Health 2013;16(3):68.

88. Hanson RK, Yates PM. Psychological treatment of sex offenders. Curr Psychiatry Rep 2013;15(3):348.

89. Meston C, Frolich PF. The neurobiology of sexual function. Arch Gen Psychiatry 2000;57:1012–30.

90. Booth BD. How to select pharmacologic treatments to manage recidivism risk in sex offenders. Curr Psychiatry 2009;8(10):60–72.

91. Bradford JM, Fedoroff P, Firestone P. Sexual violence and the clinician. [References]. In: Simon RI, Tardiff K, editors. Textbook of violence assessment and management. Arlington (VA): American Psychiatric Publishing; 2008. p. 441–60.

92. Bourget D, Bradford JM. Evidential basis for the assessment and treatment of sex offenders. Brief Treat Crisis Interv 2008;8(1):130–46.

93. Kafka MP. The monoamine hypothesis for the pathophysiology of paraphilic disorders: an update. Ann N Y Acad Sci 2003;989:86–94 [discussion: 144–53].

94. Krueger RB, Kaplan MS. Behavioral and psychopharmacological treatment of the paraphilic and hypersexual disorders. J Psychiatr Pract 2002;8(1):21–32.

95. Bradford JM. The neurobiology, neuropharmacology, and pharmacological treatment of the paraphilias and compulsive sexual behaviour. Can J Psychiatry 2001;46(1):26–34.

96. Jespersen AF, Lalumière ML, Seto MC. Sexual abuse history among adult sex offenders and non-sex offenders: a meta-analysis. Child Abuse Negl 2009; 33(3):179–92.

97. Booth BD. Elderly sexual offenders. Curr Psychiatry Rep 2016;18(4):34.

98. De Smet S, Van Hecke N, Verte D, et al. Treatment and control: a qualitative study of older mentally ill offenders' perceptions on their detention and care trajectory. Int J Offender Ther Comp Criminol 2015;59(9):964–85.

99. Sapers H. 41st annual report of the Office of the Correctional Investigator 2013-2014. Ottawa (Canada): Her Majesty the Queen in Right of Canada; 2014.

100. Hanson RK. Does Static-99 predict recidivism among older sexual offenders? Sex Abuse 2006;18(4):343–55.

101. Hanson RK. Age and sexual recidivism: a comparison of rapists and child molesters. Ottawa (Canada): Public Works and Government Services Canada; 2001.

102. Van Wijk AP, Blokland AA, Duits N, et al. Relating psychiatric disorders, offender and offence characteristics in a sample of adolescent sex offenders and non-sex offenders. Crim Behav Ment Health 2007;17(1):15–30.

103. Kafka MP, Prentky RA. Attention-deficit/hyperactivity disorder in males with paraphilias and paraphilia-related disorders: a comorbidity study. J Clin Psychiatry 1998;59(7):388–96.

104. Lichtenstein P, Halldner L, Zetterqvist J, et al. Medication for attention deficit–hyperactivity disorder and criminality. N Engl J Med 2012;367(21):2006–14.

105. Kafka MP, Hennen J. Psychostimulant augmentation during treatment with selective serotonin reuptake inhibitors in men with paraphilias and paraphilia-related disorders: a case series. J Clin Psychiatry 2000;61(9):664–70.

106. Marshall WL, Marshall LE. The utility of the random controlled trial for evaluating sexual offender treatment: the gold standard or an inappropriate strategy? Sex Abuse 2007;19(2):175–91.
107. Seto MC, Marques JK, Harris GT, et al. Good science and progress in sex offender treatment are intertwined: a response to Marshall and Marshall (2007). Sex Abuse 2008;20(3):247–55.

Violence by Parents Against Their Children
Reporting of Maltreatment Suspicions, Child Protection, and Risk in Mental Illness

Miranda McEwan, PhD, Susan Hatters Friedman, MD*

KEYWORDS

- Child abuse • Child maltreatment • Child neglect • Depression • Schizophrenia
- Mental illness

KEY POINTS

- Child abuse is not uncommon and has long-term detrimental effects.
- In America, physicians including psychiatrists are legally mandated to report suspicions of child abuse.
- Almost one-half of patients with serious mental illness are parents, and psychiatrists should ask about parenting.
- Studies that purport to demonstrate a higher risk of child maltreatment by parents with mental illness often have methodologic limitations.
- Mental illness should be treated, and should be considered a dynamic risk factor rather than a static risk factor when considering risk toward children.

INTRODUCTION

Psychiatrists often treat parents who are suffering from mental illness. It is often suggested that mental illness leads to child abuse or neglect. However, the risk of violence or neglect is decreased by appropriate treatment of symptoms and support. When there is a reasonable suspicion of child abuse, the psychiatrist is a mandated reporter, like other physicians are. Removing children from their parents is only one option considered by Child Protective Services (CPS) when determining a safe disposition for children they serve.

Disclosures: None.
Department of Psychological Medicine, University of Auckland, Room 12.003, Level 12, Auckland Hospital Support Building, Grafton, Auckland 1142, New Zealand
* Corresponding author.
E-mail addresses: sh.friedman@auckland.ac.nz; susanhfmd@hotmail.com

Abbreviations	
CAPTA	Child Abuse Protection and Treatment Act
CPS	Child Protective Services

DEFINITION OF CHILD ABUSE

According to the Federal Child Abuse Protection and Treatment Act (CAPTA) (42 U.S.C.A. § 5106g), as amended by the CAPTA Reauthorization Act of 2010, child abuse and neglect are a minimum set of acts defined as:

- "Any recent act or failure to act on the part of a parent or caretaker which results in death, serious physical or emotional harm, sexual abuse or exploitation"; or
- "An act or failure to act which presents an imminent risk of serious harm."

Although CAPTA includes specific definitions of sexual abuse and failure to provide appropriate medical treatment, it does not include specific definitions of neglect, physical abuse, or emotional abuse. Each state defines child maltreatment within civil and criminal statutes, with varying tolerance for "corporal punishment." Most states recognize 4 major types of maltreatment: neglect, physical abuse, sexual abuse, and emotional abuse/emotional neglect (**Table 1**). Witnessing domestic violence is defined as a type of abuse or neglect in some state laws.

Table 1
Types of maltreatment, their definition and prevalence

Type of Maltreatment	Definition[a]	Prevalence
Physical abuse	Intentional use of force against a child that results in, or has the potential to result in, an injury.[1]	*Official:* 119,517 reported cases of physical abuse (including duplicate reports for the same child); 17% of maltreatment victims.[2] 1.6 cases per 1000 children.[2] *Self-report:* 3.5%–16.7% per year.[3]
Neglect	Failure by a caregiver to meet a child's basic physical, emotional, medical/dental or educational needs.[1]	*Official:* 526,744 reported cases; 74% of maltreatment victims[2]; 7 cases per 1000 children. *Self-report:* 1.4% of children per year.[4]
Sexual abuse	Any attempted or completed sexual act, sexual contact with, or sexual exploitation of a child by a caregiver.[1]	*Official:* 58,105 reported cases; 8% of maltreatment victims[2]; 7.8 per 10,000 children. *Self-report:* Childhood prevalence of any sexual abuse 8.7% for boys, 25.3% for girls.[5]
Emotional abuse	Intentional caregiver behavior that conveys to a child that they are worthless, flawed, unloved, or valued only in meeting another's needs.[1]	*Official:* 42,290 reported cases; 6% of maltreatment victims[2]; 5.8 per 10,000 children. *Self-report:* 10.3% of children per year.[4]
Total maltreatment		*Official:* 702,208 individual victims; 9.4 for every 1000 children.[2]

[a] Definitions are based on the Centers for Disease Control and Prevention report, 2014.

During the 2014 financial year, American CPS agencies received 3.6 million referrals regarding 6.6 million children.[2] During this period, there were 702,000 estimated victims of abuse and neglect, a rate of 9.4 victims for every 1000 children.[2] Three-quarters (74%) of these children suffered neglect, 17% physical abuse, and 8.3% were sexually abused.[2] The majority of children (86%) experienced a single category of maltreatment (although they may have experienced that type of maltreatment several times). The remaining 14% were reported with more than 1 type of abuse.[2] One or both parents were the perpetrator in 91% of cases; this included the mother in 40% of cases.[2]

The prevalence of child abuse can be derived from studies using retrospective victim self-reports or survey participation, parental surveys, or statistics from official agencies. Each of these methods has flaws. In general, official rates are one-tenth the rates derived from other methods.[6] One study using latent class methods found that the likely true rate of sexual abuse was twice that which was reported.[7] A review of 66 international studies found that the prevalence of severe parental violence ranged from 3.5% to 16.7% per year.[3] An American study using self-reports found an annual prevalence of emotional abuse of 10.3% and of neglect, 1.4%.[4] A metaa-nalysis of worldwide studies of sexual abuse estimated a childhood prevalence rate of 8.7% for boys and 25.3% for girls for any type of sexual abuse.[5] In summary, the prevalence of abuse calculated using cases that are reported through official channels tend to underestimate rates of all types of maltreatment significantly, when compared with later self-report.

MANDATORY REPORTING OF SUSPICION OF ABUSE

In 48 states, mental health professionals are one specific group that are mandated to report their suspicion of child maltreatment to an appropriate agency; in New Jersey and Wyoming, all persons are required to report.[8] In America, health professionals contribute to 8% of reports to CPS.[9] The circumstances under which a mandatory reporter must make a report varies between states. Generally, a report must be made if the health professional (in their official capacity) suspects or has reason to believe that a child has been abused or neglected.[8] Another standard is that the reporter has observed or has knowledge of conditions that could reasonably result in harm to the child.[8] In Minnesota, it is mandatory to report any suspected abuse that has happened in the prior 3 years and any threat of abuse.[8] In sum, 28 states require the report of a suspicion including 11 states with wording regarding a reasonable cause to suspect. The other 22 states require reporting of a belief about abuse.[10] All jurisdictions have provisions in their statutes to maintain the confidentiality of abuse and neglect records and to protect the identity of the reporter.[8]

There is an historical shortfall of approximately 10-fold between the prevalence of child maltreatment and reporting to child protection agencies.[6] As noted, retrospective self-report studies of child abuse victimization find substantially higher rates than what is reported by physicians.[10] In 1 prospective study, although doctors attending injured children suspected abuse in 10% of the cases that they saw, only 6% were reported.[11] Clinicians reported 73% of cases that they considered likely or very likely to be abuse, but only 24% of children where they considered abuse "possible."[11] Severe injuries were more likely to be reported, particularly if the injury was not consistent with the given history or the child's developmental level.[11] Indeed, experts may interpret their duty to report differently depending on the severity of injuries, which is a risky practice.[10] Other studies have demonstrated variations in both whether doctors suspected abuse and how certain about maltreatment doctors feel that they need to be, before reporting to CPS.[10]

A further analysis found that clinicians' likelihood of reporting suspected maltreatment was influenced by: familiarity with the family and their circumstances including knowledge of previous CPS involvement, inconsistencies in the history, mechanism of injury, and delays in seeking treatment.[12] Clinicians who did not report their suspicions of maltreatment described that they had consulted with colleagues or other resources, and were more likely to believe that reporting their suspicions would result in an adverse outcome for the child and their family.[12] Although clinicians may be concerned that their suspicions lack adequate basis, legally they are required to report any reasonable suspicion.[8] Importantly, if a report of abuse is made in good faith, then mandated reporters have immunity from civil or criminal liability under state laws.

The shortfall between the prevalence of maltreatment and report to child protection agencies is compounded by the small proportion of reports which are substantiated. Only one-quarter (26%) of cases reach the threshold for substantiation of maltreatment in the United States.[2] The remaining three-quarters (74%) of cases may have insufficient evidence, poor family cooperation with the investigation, or the service being unable to investigate owing to lack of CPS personnel or resources, or there may have been a lack of maltreatment.[2]

Despite several studies showing higher rates of allegations of maltreatment, a recent review of the literature did not find any study that investigated recognition of child maltreatment as part of the care of parents who were accessing mental health services.[9,13]

PSYCHIATRISTS AS REPORTERS

Psychiatrists are mandated reporters of child abuse, yet are often reluctant to breach confidentiality. Therapists who do not report are most commonly concerned with the loss of the treatment alliance with the potentially abusive parent. However, compliance with mandatory reporting in many cases "contributes positively to the therapeutic process."[14] Despite limited research, in one study, Watson and Levine found that one-half of reports of child abuse were filed during the first 3 months of therapy.[14] In most cases, reporting did not ruin or significantly harm the therapeutic alliance with the parent, although almost one-quarter (24%) did terminate treatment after a report was considered or filed. Watson and Levine considered[14]

> it is possible … that it is trust, not absolute confidentiality that is essential for the psychotherapeutic relationship. Trust may develop or be maintained even though confidentiality can not be guaranteed or has been breached; clients can accept the disclosure of confidential communications if they feel that the therapist has no choice under the law.

Reports to CPS are generally made by phone (**Table 2**). CPS have the goals of keeping families together where possible, and ensuring a safe environment for children. CPS investigates reports, may initiate court actions, offers referral to parenting classes and additional supports for families in need. It should generally be discussed with the patient that one is mandated to report, and the benefits of CPS involvement, rather than only potential negative consequences of which they are already likely aware.

Reports should be made to CPS when there is a reasonable suspicion of abuse, neglect, or of significant risk to the child. As well, cases of denial or concealment of pregnancy without prenatal care may be reported for potential concerns of neglect—the mother who may not have even recognized that she is pregnant for

Table 2
Helpful websites regarding child maltreatment and protection

Website	Description
https://www.childwelfare.gov	Gateway for official information produced by the US Department of Health & Human Services, Administration for Children & Families and the Children's Bureau. • Federal and state definitions of maltreatment and requirements for mandatory reporting. • Resources for recognising, preventing, and responding to child abuse and neglect. • Information about supporting and preserving families and services available. • Information about immunity for reporting in good faith.
http://www.cdc.gov/violenceprevention/childmaltreatment/	Administered by the Centers for Disease Control and Prevention. • Focus on child abuse and neglect prevention. • Information about risk and protective factors, prevention strategies. • Data on prevalence of child maltreatment.
http://www.aacap.org/aacap/families_and_youth/resource_centers/Child_Abuse_Resource_Center/Home.aspx	Website of the American Academy of Child & Adolescent Psychiatry, child abuse resource center. • Resources for youth, family and clinicians about abuse and treatment.
https://www.childhelp.org/story-resource-center/child-abuse-education-prevention-resources/	Website run by Childhelp foundation • Resources about child abuse prevention and education. • Online resources and literary resources for children to prevent abuse or help recovery from abuse.
http://www.nccafv.org/child_abuse_reporting_numbers_co.htm	Child abuse reporting numbers by state

9 months suddenly has responsibility for a newborn infant. These mothers frequently retain custody.[15]

In addition to reporting, psychiatric hospitalization should be considered if the risk stems from active symptoms of mental illness. Emergency hospitalization (civil commitment) should be considered in cases where there is serious risk to others (including a child) owing to mental illness. As well, hospitalization should be strongly considered in cases where there is concern about risk of infanticide owing to acute mental illness symptoms—for example, suicidal depression in a loving mother or postpartum psychosis with delusions about the child (for a fuller discussion, see Friedman and Resnick[16]).

PARENTS WITH MENTAL ILLNESS

Mental health professionals do not always ask if their patients are parents.[17,18] A survey of psychiatrists found that 69% asked their female patients if they were mothers 90% to 100% of the time, and 10% asked less than one-third of the time or never.[17] Yet, one-half of women with serious mental illness are parents[19] and 10% to 20% of women with serious mental illness are actively parenting dependent children in their home.[20,21]

Between 5% and 30% of children have a parent afflicted with mental illness, and 3% to 6% have a parent with serious drug misuse.[22]

In the postpartum period, women are at greater risk for new or recurrent serious mental illness, particularly mood disorders. Parents with limited insight into their mental illness are more likely to cause harm to their children.[23] However, symptoms of mental illness are often transient and responsive to treatment and are, therefore, not indicative of overall parenting ability.[24]

About one-half of parents with schizophrenia lose custody of their children.[25] Overall, one-quarter of mothers with serious mental illness lose custody.[26] Fear of custody loss leads to a decrease in disclosure of parenting difficulties in mothers with serious mental illness[27] and may also decrease help-seeking behaviors.

IS MENTAL ILLNESS A RISK FACTOR FOR CHILD MALTREATMENT?

Parental mental illness is often considered a major risk factor for violence against children. In reality, most parents with mental illness do not abuse their children, and most parents who abuse their children are not mentally ill. Despite a dearth of literature, the idea that all persons with mental illness are at risk of child maltreatment is a prevalent view. This implies that, considering the frequency of mental illness (by the various definitions used in the various studies), approximately one-half of the population is considered at increased risk for abusing their children.

A qualitative study of 40 parents with serious mental illness, their children, and social workers involved in their care found no evidence of physical harm or neglect and, although the children had taken on some responsibilities of caring for their parents, this was often seen as positive by both the parent and the child.[28] In this study, it was suggested that there was a lack of parental support from mental health teams and a lack of recognition interventions should be targeted to helping the family work as a unit.[28] One study that measured maternal depression at 2 time points found that a reduction in depression score was associated with better parenting behaviors, better child behavior, and a decrease in child psychopathology.[29]

Mental illness in a woman appears to increase the risk of victimization by intimate partner violence.[30] Since witnessing domestic violence is conceptualized as child abuse in some states, this may contribute to reports of child abuse for mothers with mental illness.

If one considers which symptoms may lead to child maltreatment, it may be the negative symptoms or disorganized thinking of schizophrenia, which leads to neglect, for example. Paranoia or hallucinations could precipitate violence. Low energy and motivation in depression may lead to neglect, similarly to leading to poor self-care. Irritability, impulsivity, poor judgment, and the reckless behaviors of mania may lead to abuse or neglect. Importantly, treatment diminishes symptoms, and one would expect treatment to be protective as it is for other types of violence. Thus, risk of child maltreatment from mental illness should be considered as a dynamic rather than as a static risk.

We suggest that, although symptomatic mental illness may be associated with maltreatment, parents who have been diagnosed with mental illness and treated effectively, in the absence of substance misuse, personality disorder, are not at higher risk of maltreating their children. Although substance abuse and personality disorders may be comorbidities of serious mental illness, they should be considered separately as risk factors among individual parents.

Many studies that purportedly demonstrate that the risk of perpetrating maltreatment is higher among with parents with mental illness have major methodologic limitations. For example, studies have used varying definitions of mental illness itself, including not only serious mental illness (bipolar disorder, schizophrenia, recurrent major depression) but even including substance use disorders, self-reported depressive symptoms, personality issues, and posttraumatic stress disorder. For example, The National Institute of Mental Health Epidemiologic Catchment Area study found that 58% of those who reported having ever abused a child had been diagnosed with a psychiatric illness during their lifetime; however, excluding antisocial personality disorder, they found that less than 5% of their subjects with mental health disorders had abused or neglected children.[31]

Furthermore, studies may not consider whether the mental illness was treated or untreated, in remission, or whether the parent was acutely unwell. As well, verified child maltreatment is not always an outcome measure. Studies may rely on self-report alone, and retrospective studies may demonstrate recall bias. For example, 1 study found that psychopathology and a personal history of childhood abuse were correlated independently with an increase in child abuse even after controlling for demographics and family of origin characteristics.[32] Both this and the aforementioned National Institute of Mental Health Epidemiologic Catchment Area study assessed the existence and extent of child abuse retrospectively and by self-report, without collateral evidence or documentation. It has been suggested that parents with psychological problems may actually be more likely to report child maltreatment when it occurs, compared with their mentally healthy counterparts, increasing the apparent correlation between parental mental health and child abuse. In addition, the studies used "lifetime diagnosis of a psychiatric disorder" and abuse or neglect of a child at some point during their life. Neither study investigated whether the parent was symptomatic or receiving treatment before or concurrent with the abuse.[31,32]

Even the well-designed Avon Longitudinal Study of Parents and Children[33] demonstrated some of these issues. They found that parental psychiatric history correlated with higher risk. Psychiatric history, however, included psychiatric illness even before pregnancy, and antenatal questionnaires were used to inquire about depression, substance/alcohol abuse and other. As well, however, the measure was of investigation or registration on the child protection register, and thus not necessarily substantiated abuse. Similarly, a recent study of predictors among military parents[34] used the risk of maltreatment as assessed by the Child Abuse Potential Inventory, rather than actual child mistreatment, as an outcome. The Child Abuse Potential Inventory is meant to measure a parent's potential for abuse.[35] Some studies have used this index as a proxy for child maltreatment. However, one of the items on the index is "unhappiness." Therefore, those with depression would be expected to score higher on this index, and of course, will seem to have a higher risk.

In a recent reanalysis of the MacArthur violence risk database, we calculated the prevalence of acts of violence toward children committed by 2 cohorts. We compared those who had been diagnosed with a serious mental illness and were recently discharged from a psychiatric hospital with community controls who were matched for age, gender, and socioeconomic status. Violence was self-reported, but also included interviews of collateral informants and court or police reports. Serious mental illness was defined as including schizophrenia, psychotic disorders, bipolar disorder, and recurrent depression. We found that parents with severe mental illness that was treated were not at an increased risk of violence toward a child, compared with their community counterparts.[13] Psychiatric care thus may be protective against child maltreatment.

SUMMARY

Stigmatizing mental illness may lead to lower rates of help-seeking behavior among parents experiencing symptoms of mental illness, for fear of loss of custody. Rather, the large number of parents with mental illness need support, understanding, and encouragement to continue in their treatment. Substance abuse is a known serious and independent risk factor for all kinds of violence. Yet, often, studies lump together serious mental illness with substance abuse. Studies that purport to demonstrate additional risk of child maltreatment from these parents based on them having mental illness often have serious methodologic issues. Some examples of the methodologic issues found in child abuse/mental illness studies include their often retrospective nature, relying on memories of past abuse; vague definitions of mental illness without consideration of treatment; vague definitions of maltreatment, which may include mere suspicion of abuse rather than verification; and some rely on self-report of maltreatment. When psychiatrists have a reasonable suspicion of child maltreatment, CPS should be contacted, to protect children.

REFERENCES

1. Leeb RT, National Center for Injury Prevention and Control (U.S.). Child maltreatment surveillance: uniform definitions for public health and recommended data elements. 1st edition. Atlanta (GA): Centers for Disease Control and Prevention; National Center for Injury Prevention and Control; 2008. p. viii, 135.
2. U.S. Department of Health & Human Services, Administration of Children, Youth and Families, Children's Bureau. Child maltreatment 2014. 2016.
3. Woodman J, Pitt M, Wentz R, et al. Performance of screening tests for child physical abuse in accident and emergency departments. Health Technol Assess 2008;12(33):1–95.
4. Finkelhor D, Ormrod R, Turner H, et al. The victimization of children and youth: a comprehensive, national survey. Child Maltreat 2005;10(1):5–25.
5. Andrews G, Corry J, Slade T, et al. Child sexual abuse: comparative quantification of health risks. Geneva (Switzerland): World Health Organisation; 2004.
6. Gilbert R, Widom CS, Browne K, et al. Burden and consequences of child maltreatment in high-income countries. Lancet 2009;373(9657):68–81.
7. Fergusson DM, Horwood LJ, Woodward LJ. The stability of child abuse reports: a longitudinal study of the reporting behaviour of young adults. Psychol Med 2000; 30(3):529–44.
8. Child Welfare Information Gateway. Mandatory reporters of child abuse and neglect. Washington, DC: U.S. Department of Health & Human Services; 2016.
9. Gilbert R, Kemp A, Thoburn J, et al. Recognising and responding to child maltreatment. Lancet 2009;373(9658):167–80.
10. Levi BH, Portwood SG. Reasonable suspicion of child abuse: finding a common language. J Law Med Ethics 2011;39(1):62–9.
11. Flaherty EG, Sege RD, Griffith J, et al. From suspicion of physical child abuse to reporting: primary care clinician decision-making. Pediatrics 2008;122(3):611–9.
12. Jones R, Flaherty EG, Binns HJ, et al. Clinicians' description of factors influencing their reporting of suspected child abuse: report of the Child Abuse Reporting Experience Study Research Group. Pediatrics 2008;122(2):259–66.
13. Friedman SH, McEwan MV. Risk assessments for violence by parents towards children. Ft Lauderdale (FL): American Academy of Psychiatry and the Law Annual Meeting; 2015.

14. Watson H, Levine M. Psychotherapy and mandated reporting of child abuse. Am J Orthopsychiatry 1989;59(2):246–56.

15. Friedman SH, Heneghan A, Rosenthal M. Characteristics of women who do not seek prenatal care and implications for prevention. J Obstet Gynecol Neonatal Nurs 2009;38(2):174–81.

16. Friedman SH, Resnick PJ. Child murder by mothers: patterns and prevention. World Psychiatry 2007;6(3):137–41.

17. Friedman SH, Sorrentino RM, Stankowski JE, et al. Psychiatrists' knowledge about maternal filicidal thoughts. Compr Psychiatry 2008;49(1):106–10.

18. DeChillo N, Matorin S, Hallahan C. Children of psychiatric patients: rarely seen or heard. Health Soc Work 1987;12(4):296–302.

19. Royal College of Psychiatrists. Parents as patients: supporting the needs of patients who are parents and their children. In: College Report, 2011.

20. Blanch AK, Nicholson J, Purcell J. Parents with severe mental illness and their children: the need for human services integration. J Ment Health Adm 1994; 21(4):388–96.

21. White CL, Nicholson J, Fisher WH, et al. Mothers with severe mental illness caring for children. J Nerv Ment Dis 1995;183(6):398–403.

22. Advisory Council on the Misuse of Drugs. Hidden Harm: responding to the needs of children of problem drug users. London (United Kingdom): Home Office; 2003.

23. Mullick M, Miller LJ, Jacobsen T. Insight into mental illness and child maltreatment risk among mothers with major psychiatric disorders. Psychiatr Serv 2001;52(4): 488–92.

24. Jacobsen T, Miller LJ. Mentally ill mothers who have killed: three cases addressing the issue of future parenting capability. Psychiatr Serv 1998;49(5):650–7.

25. Seeman MV. Intervention to prevent child custody loss in mothers with schizophrenia. Schizophr Res Treatment 2012;2012:796763.

26. Hollingsworth LD. Child custody loss among women with persistent severe mental illness. Soc Work Res 2004;28(4):199–209.

27. Diaz-Caneja A, Johnson S. The views and experiences of severely mentally ill mothers–a qualitative study. Soc Psychiatry Psychiatr Epidemiol 2004;39(6): 472–82.

28. Aldridge J. The experiences of children living with and caring for parents with mental illness. Child Abuse Rev 2006;15:79–88.

29. Shaw DS, Connell A, Dishion TJ, et al. Improvements in maternal depression as a mediator of intervention effects on early childhood problem behavior. Dev Psychopathol 2009;21(2):417–39.

30. Friedman SH, Loue S. Incidence and prevalence of intimate partner violence by and against women with severe mental illness. J Womens Health (Larchmt) 2007; 16(4):471–80.

31. Egami Y, Ford DE, Greenfield SF, et al. Psychiatric profile and sociodemographic characteristics of adults who report physically abusing or neglecting children. Am J Psychiatry 1996;153(7):921–8.

32. Medley A, Sachs-Ericsson N. Predictors of parental physical abuse: the contribution of internalizing and externalizing disorders and childhood experiences of abuse. J Affect Disord 2009;113(3):244–54.

33. Sidebotham P, Golding J, ALSPAC Study Team. Avon Longitudinal Study of Parents and Children. Child maltreatment in the "children of the nineties" a longitudinal study of parental risk factors. Child Abuse Negl 2001;25(9): 1177–200.

34. Schaeffer CM, Alexander P, Bethke K, et al. Predictors of child abuse potential among military parents: comparing mothers and fathers. J Fam Violence 2005; 20(2):123–9.
35. Robertson KR, Milner JS. Construct validity of the child abuse potential inventory. J Clin Psychol 1983;39(3):426–9.

Gender Considerations in Violence

Renee Sorrentino, MD[a],*, Susan Hatters Friedman, MD[b], Ryan Hall, MD[c]

KEYWORDS

- Violence • Gender • Women • Intimate partner violence • Risk assessment
- Female stalkers • Gender bias

KEY POINTS

- Women account for a minority of the incarcerated population. However, the rate of incarceration in women is increasing.
- Women are much less likely to be convicted of a violence offense compared with men.
- Both women and men share the following risk factors for violence: younger age, a history of childhood conduct problems, substance use, and legal history.
- The gender disparity in violence decreases in the setting of mental illness.
- Some differences in female sex offenders are higher rates of abuse compared with men, increased likelihood of victimizing biological children, and greater likelihood of engaging in a sexual offense with a codefendant.
- Women who kill their children most often do so in the context of chronic abuse or neglect.
- Like men, women may be violent in intimate partner relationships and they have various reasons and motives.

INTRODUCTION

Although women account for only 7% of the incarcerated population, the number is growing.[1] Men are more likely to commit acts of violence. However, this may not be true in all settings. Studies have indicated that the gender difference in violence decreases in the setting of mental illness.[2] Understanding the gender differences and similarities in violent behaviors helps to establish accurate risk assessment and treatment. The application of gender-informed risk assessments might be instrumental in reducing the risk of future violent behaviors. The role of gender in risk assessment,

Disclosures: The authors have nothing to disclose.
[a] Department of Psychiatry, Harvard School of Medicine, 15 Parkman Street, Boston, MA 02114, USA; [b] Department of Psychological Medicine, University of Auckland, Auckland Hospital Support Building, Room 12-003, Grafton, Auckland, New Zealand; [c] Department of Psychiatry, University of Central Florida College of Medicine, University of South Florida, Barry University Dwayne O. Andreas School of Law, 2500 West Lake Mary Boulevard, Lake Mary, FL 32746, USA
* Corresponding author.
E-mail address: rsorrentino@partners.org

sexual offending, intimate partner violence, and child murder is explored in this article.

RISK ASSESSMENT IN WOMEN

Violence risk instruments assign a classification for the likelihood that an individual will commit violence (low, moderate, or high risk). Many of these instruments were primarily normed on male prison populations,[3] which has led to debate in the literature about whether certain static factors among men (eg, the sex of the victim) accurately predict the likelihood of female-perpetrated violence or reoffense.[3–5] However, some research suggests that certain risk factors found among men apply to women as well.[3,4,6,7] For example, violence is more likely to be committed by younger individuals whether male or female.[3,4,6,7] Similarly, a history of conduct problems as a child, substance use, and legal history are all risk factors that apply to both men and women.[3,4,6,7] In addition, there may be specific risk factors for women that assessment instruments do not measure, such as being a victim of intimate partner violence (**Box 1**). For example, an epidemiologic study done about British women in the community found the following to be the strongest factors for predicting future violence among women: young age, residence in social-assisted housing, history of early conduct problems, being a victim of intimate partner violence, having a history of self-harm behaviors, excessive drinking, and past criminal justice involvement.[4]

An additional confounding variable for violence risk assessment is mental health history. For example, incarcerated populations often have co-occurring diagnoses such as personality disorders, PTSD, and substance use disorders. When developing assessment instruments, co-occurring diagnoses may cause skewed results compared with the results produced by a general population sample or a sample showing a single disease state such as depression.[8] For example, in a recent large Swedish study, Fazel and colleagues[9] sought to determine the risk of violent crimes among patients with a recent outpatient diagnosis of depression. As part of the study, the investigators considered an outpatient population diagnosed with depression compared with age-matched controls. The investigators did a secondary analysis involving siblings to try to factor out environmental influences, personality disorders,

---

Box 1
Domains of risk factors for violence-prone women

Childhood adversity: foster care, runaway, unstable family structure

Conduct problems: school expulsions, juvenile offenses

Living situation: unstable housing, subsidized housing, homelessness

Relationships: dysfunctional, unstable, unmarried

Past victimization: sexual abuse, victim of intimate partner violence

Lifestyle: lifestyle that leads to frequent interactions with police or authorities

Adult trauma: victim of crime, traumatic separation

Mental health history: depression, anxiety, psychosis, self-harm attempt, personality disorders

Substance abuse

Data from Yang M, Wong SC, Coid JW. Violence, mental health and violence risk factors among community women: an epidemiological study based on two national household surveys in the UK. BMC Public Health 2013;12:1020.

substance use, violence history, and income levels. Violence was determined based on conviction in the Swedish court system for a violent crime in which there was no plea of not guilty by reason of insanity, and 0.5% of the depressed women committed a violent offense compared with 0.2% of the nondepressed women (odds ratio [OR], 2.8; 95% confidence interval [CI], 2.3–3.3). The rate for depressed men was 3.7%, so depressed women were less likely to be violent than their depressed male counterparts. In review of all the factors associated with a violent crime, this study replicated what many other studies have found: that the most important factors for risk of violence are a history of past violent acts and substance use for both men and women.

Note that Fazel and colleagues[10] obtained similar results in a comparable study about violent outcomes among individuals with schizophrenia and other related disorders (eg, delusional disorder, schizoaffective disorder, unspecified psychosis) in a Swedish population over age 38. Again the conclusion was that a mental health diagnosis increased the risk for violence for both men and women, especially for individuals with a history of a substance use disorder, criminal behavior, and self-harm attempts. In this study, 2.7% of the women with schizophrenia and other related disorders and 10.7% of the men committed a violent crime within 5 years of being diagnosed. This incidence resulted in an adjusted OR for women with schizophrenia compared with the general population of 14.9 (95% CI, 13.2–16.8). An additional finding of the study is the effect of societal change on the incidences of violence. The investigators found that as the number of days of inpatient hospitalization decreased from the 1970s to the late 2000s, the incidence of violence increased (OR, 5.6%; 95% CI, 2.6%-8.4%; adjusted OR for substances, 5.0%; 95% CI, 1.9% to 7.9%). These results raise the question of how treatment conditions and changes in such conditions over time may affect violence risk assessment. Most of the individuals who committed violent acts were between the ages of 25 and 44 years, and this was consistent with other studies about violence, which found that younger people commit violent acts. However, given the population studied, the correlation between violence and young age may also be related to the phenomenon of positive symptoms of psychosis (eg, hallucinations, delusions) declining with increasing age, resulting in the negative symptoms such as avoidance becoming more prominent over the lifespan of the individual, thus decreasing the risk of violent offenses over time.[11]

It should also be noted that a potential limitation of both the Fazel and colleagues[9,10] studies is that they did not factor in whether the individuals with the diagnoses of depression or schizophrenia received appropriate treatment (eg, whether they accessed appropriate treatment, the frequency of visits, the type of therapy, and doses of medications), or complied with treatment (eg, whether they filled prescriptions or attended appointments). This is important because the MacArthur Study of mental disorder and violence previously found that individuals with mental illness, if complaint with treatment, were at no greater risk of committing violence than the general population.[12] The rates reported may only be applicable to populations or health systems with a similar rate of use and treatment to those in Sweden. However, with regard to the context of this article, the research shows that there is a gender difference for the rate of violence that is mediated by mental illness, even if it may be caused more by confounding factors (eg, whether women are more like to obtain treatment or be compliant with treatment of mental illness) than true disease-state differences between genders. As noted in a recent Australian study by Harris and colleagues,[13] men with affective, anxiety, or substance use disorders were less likely to seek treatment over a

1-year period compared with women with the same conditions (aOR, 0.46; 95% CI, 0.30–0.70).[10]

FEMALE SEX OFFENDERS

Female sex offenders are a poorly understood group. Most sex offender research has been about men. The dearth of research about female sex offenders has resulted in the application of evaluation, treatment, and risk prediction principles from the male sex offender literature. To date, there is insufficient evidence to support the use of male sex offender data for women. Studies estimate that women comprise between 1% and 5% of the total sex offender population.[14,15] National statistics about sexual offenders show lower rates of female sex offenders, whereas victim report studies show higher percentages of female offenders.[16] International studies based on victimization surveys and official records from Canada, the United Kingdom, the United States, Australia, and New Zealand found that women make up 5% of all sexual offenders.[17,18] As with male sex offenders, it is difficult to estimate the true prevalence of female sex offenders. Uniquely, for women, there are cultural and societal stereotypes of women being incapable and uninterested in sexual offending. This stereotype undoubtedly affects the accurate identification of female sex offenders. When female sex offending occurs, it is often perceived as less harmful compared with male offending, or perceived to be initiated by a man. Victims of female perpetrators may be more reluctant to report the abuse because of the relationship with the perpetrator, which is commonly incestuous, as well as the societal perception of women as caretakers and nurturing. However, bias exists in the detection of sexual offenders and is not limited to the general public. The medical and law enforcement communities share the traditional preconception of women as nonviolent nurturers. Biased physicians and police officers do not detect sexual offenses perpetrated by women. As a result, those professions, which could have a role in the detection and prevention of sexual abuse, are not playing that role.

The female sex offender research has identified characteristics of offenders and victim variables.[19] Offender histories of childhood sexual abuse and intimate partner victimization violence are consistently supported in the literature. Female offenders report abuse histories at an earlier age than male offenders, and experience a longer duration of abuse, greater severity, and higher rates of incest and rape.[20,21] Female sex offenders, like female nonsexual offenders, have high rates of psychiatric disorders. Female sex offenders report high rates of mood, anxiety, and substance use disorders.[20,22] Fazel and colleagues[23] found that one-third of female sex offenders had a past history of psychiatric hospitalization. Studies have not consistently found a difference in psychiatric symptoms or diagnoses when female sex offenders were compared with male offenders. Compared with the general population, female sex offenders have higher rates of psychiatric illness. In one study, between 50% and 75% of women reported a history of intimate partner violence.[21,24] Like their male counterparts, limited social supports and intimacy deficits were common in female offenders. Female offenders, like male offenders, often show cognitive distortions or beliefs that minimize sexually abusive behavior. One of the unique replicated findings is that women are more likely than men to commit a sex offense with a male co-offender or as the result of coercion by a man.

Most victims of female sex offenders are known to the offender. Studies examining victim characteristics found that women are more likely than men to abuse their biological children or children they have cared for.[25] Women are also less discerning of gender when selecting a victim.[26] Most studies, although not all, found female sex offenders to select male and female victims equally. Most victims of female offenders are young (<18 years old), in contrast with male offender victims.[27]

Overall, male sex offenders have a more extensive criminal history and higher recidivism rate compared with women. Sexual offenses committed by women generally do not involve violent force. Rape is generally defined as penetration of an orifice by an object. Acts of rape are less common among female sex offenders, but, when they occur, the victims tend to be of the same gender, unlike the victims of male-perpetrated rapes.[28] Although studies have shown that women rarely engage in rape behavior, the prevalence may be obscured by the gender bias in sexual offending. For example, before 2012, the FBI defined rape as the "carnal knowledge of a female forcibly and against her will."[29] In recognition of this limiting defense, the FBI broadened the definition of rape to "any kind of penetration of another person, regardless of gender, without the victim's consent."[29]

There are cases of female offenders working with male coperpetrators to engage in acts of rape and sexual abuse on adult victims or sexual violence toward children. In these cases, the female offender often aided the male perpetrator. The female perpetrator often would also engage in sexual acts with the male perpetrator in front of the victim.[30] It was thought that violent female sexual abusers, especially those who engaged in acts with a male coperpetrator, were under-reported because the women often cooperated with authorities against their male partners or it was assumed by authorities that the female offender was another forced victim. Female rapists who act alone are not well defined in the literature. This group of violent female sex offenders is thought to represent the minority.

Attempts to better define female sexual offending have resulted in the classification or typology of female offenders. The typology created by Mathews and colleagues[31] (1989) is the most cited. Mathews and colleagues[31] described 3 typologies: male coerced, predisposed, and teacher/lover. The male-coerced group refers to women who depend on the male in the relationship. They have histories of sexual abuse and poor relationships. These women participate in sexual offending behavior to maintain the relationship. The predisposed group refers to women who are predisposed to sexual offending because of a history of incest, deviant sexual fantasies, and psychological difficulties. The predisposed female offenders were more likely to abuse their own children or intrafamilial victims. The last group described by Mathews and colleagues[31] is teacher/lover. Teacher/lover offenders are often in dysfunctional peer relationships and idealize a relationship with a minor. Most of these women did not consider their behavior to be criminal. Vandiver and Kercher[32] described a statistically validated typology from a study of more than 450 female sex offenders. They categorized female sex offenders into 6 groups based on the demographics of victim characteristics and criminal histories. The 6 categories were dominant woman abuse (adult woman abusing adult male), experimented/exploiter (younger offender exploiting a child under her care), babysitter abuse (younger boy assaulted by unrelated female), teacher/lover (teacher abusing student), male-coerced molester (passive offender acting with partner), and male-accompanied offender (active offender acting with partner).[32] The largest group, as in the Mathews and colleagues[31] study, was the teacher/lover category. This group represented the women who were least likely to have an arrest for a sexual assault.[32] These findings dispel the societal myth that women do not commit sexual offenses because of their maternal proclivity to nurture. Rather, it is these women who are in nurturing relationships who may commit sexual offenses.

The prevalence of paraphilic disorders among female sex offenders is not known. Most of the literature about paraphilias in women is limited to case studies and small samples. Federoff and colleagues[33] reviewed 15 female sex offenders using Diagnostic and Statistical Manual of Mental Disorders, Fourth Edition, criteria for paraphilias, and approximately half of the women met criteria for a paraphilia. The most common diagnoses were pedophilia, sexual sadism, and exhibitionism.

The prediction of sex offender recidivism among women is difficult given the low base rate and the limited research. Unlike their male counterparts, there are no validated risk assessment instruments for women. The current appraisal of risk to recidivate in women is adopted from the male literature. A study of 380 female sex offenders by Cortoni and Hanson[17] found a 5-year recidivism rate of 1%. A meta-analysis of 10 studies consisting of a total of 2490 female sex offenders found a 3% rate of recidivism over 6.5 years.[18] The empirically derived risk factors for male sexual recidivism are applied to women without validation.

Female sex offenders are rarely violent. However, estimation of the prevalence and characteristics of female sex offenders is poorly understood. Future research in the role of gender in sexual offending should begin to answer these questions.

WOMEN PERPETRATORS OF INTIMATE PARTNER VIOLENCE

Women represent approximately 14% of violent offenders. Women are most likely to be violent in the home, toward family.[34]

Intimate partner violence includes sexual, physical, and emotional abuse. Often it is dangerously conceptualized that women are merely victims, but women may alternatively be the primary aggressor in a heterosexual relationship.[35]

Violence may be bidirectional. Violence may also occur in homosexual relationships. Violence may occur because of anger, revenge, control, or either paranoid or rational self-defense.[36] Female batterers have been described as histrionic, compulsive, or narcissistic.[37] Women with severe mental illness may present as intimate partner violence victims, perpetrators, or both.[38]

Straus[39] noted that more than 200 studies have documented that similar percentages of men and women are assaultive toward their partners. Data from the Bureau of Justice Statistics reveals that, in intimate partner violence, 27% of male victims and 18% of female victims have had weapons used against them; 5% of women and 19% of men are hit with an object. It is estimated that half (50%) of female victims and 44% of men are injured by intimate partner violence, with 13% of women and 5% of men experiencing serious injury.[40]

After being discovered by the legal system, batterers often receive court orders to attend batterer intervention programs. However, these programs often presuppose a single male-oriented mechanism of violence related to a man's proprietary view of a woman. Because of the single perspective, such programs are unlikely to be effective in other populations.

Battered women's syndrome (BWS), although labeled a syndrome, is used in the legal arena rather than the medical arena as a defense for murder. BWS is based on the model of learned helplessness, in which a woman's role is that of a passive abuse victim. BWS is used to help juries understand why a woman may kill her abusive partner with excessive force, and when it did not appear to an outsider that she was in imminent danger.

When evaluating a woman in the context of intimate partner violence, clinicians should inquire about situations in which there has been violence, precipitants, aggression, and the potential for bidirectional violence.[41] If clinicians do not consider that women too may be the aggressors, then issues may not be fully investigated and violence may continue.

WOMEN WHO KILL THEIR CHILDREN

Fathers and mothers murder their children at similar rates overall. Mothers are less likely than fathers to also commit suicide at the time of the child murder.[42] In addition, in neonaticide (murder in the first day of life), the culprit is virtually always the mother.[35]

Both mothers and fathers are most likely to kill their children in the context of chronically abusing or neglecting that child.[43] This situation is very different from killing because of a psychotic motive, or in association with suicidality. It is noteworthy that fathers and mothers kill their children at similar rates because, in other types of murder, men predominate by far.

Mothers who kill their children are more likely to be shown mercy by courts than fathers who kill their children, both in America and internationally. Infanticide laws exist in 24 nations.[43] In general, infanticide laws decrease the penalty from murder to a penalty akin to that for manslaughter, only for mothers who kill their children, and usually only within the first year of life. Mothers are more likely than fathers to be found not guilty by reason of insanity for the crime of child murder.[44,45]

In light of this, it is important that psychiatrists inquire whether their patients are parents with responsibility for their minor children, because this may not always be considered.[46] Clinicians should consider the risk that mentally unwell parents may pose to their young children, as discussed elsewhere in this issue (See Miranda McEwan and Susan Hatters Friedman's article, "Violence by parents against their children"). Risk of filicide (child murder by parent) related to altruistic or altruistic psychotic motives should be considered among mentally unwell mothers. Forensic interviews after child murder by parents are discussed further elsewhere.[42]

GENDER BIAS

Gender bias, including stereotypes about gender role, sexual offending, and intimate partner violence, are pervasive in our culture. These biases potentially affect the policing of violent offenses, their legal outcomes, and the management. Studies of the role of gender in the determination of legal outcomes conclude that female defendants receive more lenient sentencing than male defendants. For example, for charges resulting from death, women are more likely than men to be incarcerated for manslaughter rather than murder.[1] Although not as extensively studied, gender bias seems to be present in sexual offending and intimate partner violence. As clinicians learn more about the relationship between gender and violence, the gender bias should be replaced by statistically derived data about the role of gender.

SUMMARY

The role of gender should be considered in violence prediction. At present, most risk prediction in general and in specific cases such as female sex offenders and intimate partner violence depends on studies in men. However, it is clear that there are specific differences in male and female behaviors that warrant tailored risk assessment tools. The future of accurate prediction of risk should begin with steps toward understanding and uncovering the gender bias in this field.

REFERENCES

1. Carson AE, Sabol WJ. Prisoners in 2011. Bureau of Justice Statistics, Office of Justice Programs. US Department of Justice; 2012.
2. Robbins PC, Monahan J, Silver E. Mental disorder, violence, and gender. Law Hum Behav 2003;27(6):561–71.

3. Friedman SH, Hall RCW, Sorrentino R. Commentary: women, violence and insanity. J Am Acad Psychiatry Law 2013;41(4):523–8.

4. Yang M, Wong SC, Coid JW. Violence, mental health and violence risk factors among community women: an epidemiological study based on two national household surveys in the UK. BMC Public Health 2013;12:1020.

5. Barbaree HE, Langton CM, Peacock EJ. The factor structure of static actuarial items: its relation to prediction. Sex Abuse 2006;18(2):207–26.

6. Siever L. Neurobiology of aggression and violence. Am J Psychiatry 2008;165(4): 429–42.

7. Patrick C. Psychophysiological correlates of aggression and violence: an integrative review. Philos Trans R Soc Lond B Biol Sci 2008;363:2543–55.

8. Friedman SH, Collier S, Hall RCW. PTSD behind bars: incarcerated women and PTSD. In: Martin C, Preedy V, Patel V, editors. Comprehensive guide to post-traumatic stress disorder. Switzerland: Springer International; 2015.

9. Fazel S, Wolf A, Chang Z, et al. Depression and violence: a Swedish population study. Lancet Psychiatry 2015;2(3):224–32.

10. Fazel S, Wolf A, Palm C, et al. Violent crime, suicide, and premature mortality in patients with schizophrenia and related disorders: a 38-year total population study in Sweden. Lancet Psychiatry 2014;1(1):44–54.

11. Swanson JW, Swartz MS, Van Dorn RA, et al. A national study of violent behavior in persons with schizophrenia. Arch Gen Psychiatry 2006;63(5):490–9.

12. Monahan J, Steadman HJ, Silver E, et al. Rethinking risk assessment: the MacArthur study of mental disorder and violence. New York: Oxford University Press; 2001.

13. Harris MG, Baxter AJ, Reavley N, et al. Gender-related patterns and determinants of recent help-seeking for past-year affective, anxiety and substance use disorder: findings from a national epidemiological survey. Epidemiol Psychiatr Sci 2015;2:1–14.

14. Gannon TA, Rose MR. Offence-related interpretative bias in female child molesters: a preliminary study. Sex Abuse 2009;21:194–207.

15. Sandler JC, Freeman NJ. Female sex offender recidivism: a large-scale empirical analysis. Sex Abuse 2009;21(4):455–73.

16. Gannon TA, Cortoni F. Female sexual offenders: theory, assessment and treatment. Chichester (United Kingdom): John Wiley; 2010.

17. Cortoni F, Hanson RK. A review of the recidivism rates of adult female sexual offenders. Research Report No. R-169. Ottawa (Canada): Correctional Service Canada; 2005.

18. Cortoni F, Hanson RK, Coache ME. The recidivism rates of female sexual offenders are low: a meta-analysis. Sex Abuse 2010;22(4):387–401.

19. Johansson-Love J, Fremouw W. Female sex offenders: a controlled comparison of offender and victim/crime characteristics. J Fam Violence 2009;24:367–76.

20. Miccio-Fonseca LC. Adult and adolescent female sex offenders: experiences compared to other female and male sex offenders. J Psychol Human Sex 2000;11(3):75–88.

21. Elliott IA, Eldridge HJ, Ashfield S, et al. Exploring risk: potential static, dynamic, protective and treatment factors in the clinical histories of female sex offenders. J Fam Violence 2010;25:595–602.

22. Steadman HJ, Osher FC, Robbins PC, et al. Prevalence of serious mental illness among jail inmates. Psychiatr Serv 2009;60:761–5.

23. Fazel S, Sjöstedt G, Grann M, et al. Sexual offending in women and psychiatric disorder: a national case-control study. Arch Sex Behav 2010;39(1):161–7.

24. Gannon TA, Rose MR, Ward T. A descriptive model of the offense process for female sexual offenders. Sex Abuse 2008;20(3):352–74.
25. West SG, Friedhman SH, Kim KD. Women accused of sex offenses: a gender-based comparison. Behav Sci Law 2011;29(5):728–40.
26. Gannon TA, Waugh G, Taylor K, et al. Women who sexually offend display three main offense styles: a re-examination of the descriptive model of female sexual offending. Sex Abuse 2014;26(3):207–24.
27. Lewis CF, Stanley CR. Women accused of sexual offenses. Behav Sci Law 2000; 18(1):73–81.
28. Bierie DM, Davis-Siegel J. Measurement matters comparing old and new definitions of rape in federal statistical reporting. Sex Abuse 2015;27(5):443–59.
29. Federal Bureau of Investigation. Crime in the united states 2013: rape. US Government, US Department of Justice. Available at: https://ucr.fbi.gov/crime-in-the-u.s/2013/crime-in-the-u.s.-2013/violent-crime/rape/rapemain_final.pdf. Accessed May 5, 2016.
30. Almond L, McManus MA, Giles S, et al. Female sex offenders: an analysis of crime scene behaviors. J Interpers Violence 2015. [Epub ahead of print].
31. Mathews R, Matthews J, Speltz K. Female sexual offenders: an exploratory study. Brandon (VT): The Safer Society Press; 1989.
32. Vandiver DM, Kercher G. Offender and victim characteristics of registered female sexual offenders in Texas: a proposed typology of female sexual offenders. Sex Abuse 2004;16(2):121–37.
33. Fedoroff PJ, Fishell A, Fedoroff B. A case series of women evaluated for paraphilic sexual disorders. Can J Hum Sex 1999;8(2):127–40.
34. Greenfeld LA, Snell T. Women offenders. Bureau of Justice Statistics Special Report, Office of Justice Programs. US Department of Justice; 2000.
35. Friedman SH. Realistic consideration of women and violence is critical. J Am Acad Psychiatry Law 2015;43(3):273–6.
36. Friedman SH, Loue S, Heaphy E, et al. Intimate partner violence perpetrated by and against Puerto Rican women with severe mental illness. Community Ment Health J 2011;47:156–63.
37. Buttell FP, Carney MM. Women who perpetrate relationship violence: moving beyond political correctness. New York: Hawthorn Press; 2005.
38. Friedman SH, Loue S. Incidence and prevalence of intimate partner violence by and against women with severe mental illness: a review. J Womens Health 2007; 16:471–80.
39. Straus MA. Blaming the messenger for the bad news about partner violence by women: the methodological, theoretical, and value basis of the purported invalidity of the conflict tactics scales. Behav Sci Law 2012;30:538–56.
40. Catalanos S. Intimate partner violence: attributes of victimization. Bureau of Justice Statistics, Office of Justice Programs. US Department of Justice; 2013.
41. Friedman SH, Stankowski J, Loue S. Intimate partner violence and the clinician. In: Simon RI, Tardiff KT, editors. Textbook of Violence Assessment and Management. Arlington (TX): American Psychiatric Publishing; 2008. p. 483–500.
42. Friedman SH, Cavney J, Resnick PJ. Child murder by parents and evolutionary psychology. Psychiatr Clin North Am 2012a;35(4):781–95.
43. Friedman SH, Resnick PJ. Child murder by mothers: patterns and prevention. World Psychiatry 2007;6(3):137–41.
44. Friedman SH, Hrouda D, Holden C, et al. Child murder committed by severely mentally ill mothers: an examination of mothers found not guilty by reason of insanity. J Forensic Sci 2005b;50(6):1466–71.

45. Friedman SH, Cavney J, Resnick P. Mothers who kill: evolutionary underpinning and law. Behav Sci Law 2012b;30:585–97.
46. Friedman SH, Sorrentino R, Stankowski JE, et al. Psychiatrists' awareness of maternal filicidal thoughts. Compr Psychiatry 2008;49(1):106–10.

Index

Note: Page numbers of article titles are in **boldface** type.

A

Acetylcholinesterase inhibitors, for persistent aggression in dementia, 549
Aggression. *See* named subtype, e.g. *Impulsive aggression.*
    classification of, 542–543
        impulsive, 542–543
        inpatient by subtype, 543
        predatory, 542–543
        psychotic, 542
    psychotic violence and, pharmacologic approach to, 544–546
Agitation, Best Practices in the Evaluation and Treatment of Agitation, 560
Aircraft homiide-suicide, research in, 640
Amygdala, characterization of, 586
    structure and function of, 586–587
        in memory and connection with emotion, 587
        in violence-associated disorders, 587
    violence-specific neural activity in fMRI processing, 587–588
Analgesics, for persistent aggression in demention, 548
Anterior cingulate cortex (ACC), in antisocial behavior, 583
    description of, 583
    in emotional regulation, 583
    in psychopathic individuals, 583–584
Antipsychotic medications, for inpatient psychotic violence and aggression, 544–545
Antisocial personality, violence and, 580
Antisocial personality disorder (APD), correlation with brain structure on MRI, 585
Antisocial subjects, activation deficit in left frontal gyrus in, 584–585
Anxiety disorders, in sex offenders, 682
Attention-deficit/hyperactivity disorder, in sex offenders, 682–683
Atypical antipsychotics, for persistent aggression in demention, 549

B

Basal ganglia, on fMRI, abnormal caudate nucleus activation in schizophrenia, 588–589
    on MRI, reduction of nucleus accumbens in psychopathy, 599
    role in regulation of behavior, 588
    structure and function of, 588
Battered women's syndrome, 706
    batterer intervention programs in, 706
Best Practices in the Evaluation and Treatment of Agitation (BETA)
Brain functioning techniques, 581
Brain imaging techniques, 581
Brain injury(ies), violence-mediating brain areas and, 580

Psychiatr Clin N Am 39 (2016) 711–721
http://dx.doi.org/10.1016/S0193-953X(16)30063-6
0193-953X/16

psych.theclinics.com

UNITED STATES POSTAL SERVICE® Statement of Ownership, Management, and Circulation (All Periodicals Publications Except Requester Publications)

1. Publication Title	2. Publication Number	3. Filing Date
PSYCHIATRIC CLINICS OF NORTH AMERICA	000 – 703	9/18/2016

4. Issue Frequency	5. Number of Issues Published Annually	6. Annual Subscription Price
MAR, JUN, SEP, DEC	4	$300.00

7. Complete Mailing Address of Known Office of Publication (Not printer) (Street, city, county, state, and ZIP+4®)

ELSEVIER INC.
360 PARK AVENUE SOUTH
NEW YORK, NY 10010-1710

Contact Person: STEPHEN R. BUSHING
Telephone (Include area code): 215-239-3688

8. Complete Mailing Address of Headquarters or General Business Office of Publisher (Not printer)

ELSEVIER INC.
360 PARK AVENUE SOUTH
NEW YORK, NY 10010-1710

9. Full Names and Complete Mailing Addresses of Publisher, Editor, and Managing Editor (Do not leave blank)

Publisher (Name and complete mailing address)

ADRIANNE BRIGIDO, ELSEVIER INC.
1600 JOHN F KENNEDY BLVD. SUITE 1800
PHILADELPHIA, PA 19103-2899

Editor (Name and complete mailing address)

LAUREN BOYLE ELSEVIER INC.
1600 JOHN F KENNEDY BLVD. SUITE 1800
PHILADELPHIA, PA 19103-2899

Managing Editor (Name and complete mailing address)

PATRICK MANLEY, ELSEVIER INC.
1600 JOHN F KENNEDY BLVD. SUITE 1800
PHILADELPHIA, PA 19103-2899

10. Owner (Do not leave blank. If the publication is owned by a corporation, give the name and address of the corporation immediately followed by the names and addresses of all stockholders owning or holding 1 percent or more of the total amount of stock. If not owned by a corporation, give the names and addresses of the individual owners. If owned by a partnership or other unincorporated firm, give its name and address as well as those of each individual owner. If the publication is published by a nonprofit organization, give its name and address.)

Full Name	Complete Mailing Address
WHOLLY OWNED SUBSIDIARY OF REED/ELSEVIER, US HOLDINGS	1600 JOHN F KENNEDY BLVD. SUITE 1800 PHILADELPHIA, PA 19103-2899

11. Known Bondholders, Mortgagees, and Other Security Holders Owning or Holding 1 Percent or More of Total Amount of Bonds, Mortgages, or Other Securities. If none, check box ► ☐ None

Full Name	Complete Mailing Address
N/A	

12. Tax Status (For completion by nonprofit organizations authorized to mail at nonprofit rates) (Check one)
The purpose, function, and nonprofit status of this organization and the exempt status for federal income tax purposes:
☐ Has Not Changed During Preceding 12 Months
☐ Has Changed During Preceding 12 Months (Publisher must submit explanation of change with this statement)

13. Publication Title	14. Issue Date for Circulation Data Below
PSYCHIATRIC CLINICS OF NORTH AMERICA	JUNE 2016

15. Extent and Nature of Circulation			Average No. Copies Each Issue During Preceding 12 Months	No. Copies of Single Issue Published Nearest to Filing Date
a. Total Number of Copies (Net press run)			461	402
b. Paid Circulation (By Mail and Outside the Mail)	(1)	Mailed Outside-County Paid Subscriptions Stated on PS Form 3541 (Include paid distribution above nominal rate, advertiser's proof copies, and exchange copies)	159	172
	(2)	Mailed In-County Paid Subscriptions Stated on PS Form 3541 (Include paid distribution above nominal rate, advertiser's proof copies, and exchange copies)	0	0
	(3)	Paid Distribution Outside the Mails Including Sales Through Dealers and Carriers, Street Vendors, Counter Sales, and Other Paid Distribution Outside USPS®	114	134
	(4)	Paid Distribution by Other Classes of Mail Through the USPS (e.g. First-Class Mail®)	0	0
c. Total Paid Distribution [Sum of 15b (1), (2), (3), and (4)]		►	273	306
d. Free or Nominal Rate Distribution (By Mail and Outside the Mail)	(1)	Free or Nominal Rate Outside-County Copies included on PS Form 3541	52	61
	(2)	Free or Nominal Rate In-County Copies Included on PS Form 3541	0	0
	(3)	Free or Nominal Rate Copies Mailed at Other Classes Through the USPS (e.g. First-Class Mail)	0	0
	(4)	Free or Nominal Rate Distribution Outside the Mail (Carriers or other means)	0	0
e. Total Free or Nominal Rate Distribution (Sum of 15d (1), (2), (3) and (4))		►	52	61
f. Total Distribution (Sum of 15c and 15e)		►	325	367
g. Copies not Distributed (See Instructions to Publishers #4 (page #3))		►	136	35
h. Total (Sum of 15f and g)		►	461	402
i. Percent Paid (15c divided by 15f times 100)			84%	83%

* If you are claiming electronic copies, go to line 16 on page 3. If you are not claiming electronic copies, skip to line 17 on page 3.

16. Electronic Copy Circulation	Average No. Copies Each Issue During Preceding 12 Months	No. Copies of Single Issue Published Nearest to Filing Date
a. Paid Electronic Copies ►	0	0
b. Total Paid Print Copies (Line 15c) + Paid Electronic Copies (Line 16a) ►	273	306
c. Total Print Distribution (Line 15f) + Paid Electronic Copies (Line 16a) ►	325	367
d. Percent Paid (Both Print & Electronic Copies) (16b divided by 16c × 100) ►	84%	83%

☒ I certify that 50% of all my distributed copies (electronic and print) are paid above a nominal price.

17. Publication of Statement of Ownership
☒ If the publication is a general publication, publication of this statement is required. Will be printed ☐ Publication not required.
in the DECEMBER 2016 issue of this publication.

18. Signature and Title of Editor, Publisher, Business Manager, or Owner

STEPHEN R. BUSHING - INVENTORY DISTRIBUTION CONTROL MANAGER

Date: 9/18/2016

I certify that all information furnished on this form is true and complete. I understand that anyone who furnishes false or misleading information on this form or who omits material or information requested on the form may be subject to criminal sanctions (including fines and imprisonment) and/or civil sanctions (including civil penalties).

PS Form **3526**, July 2014 [Page 3 of 4 (see instructions page 4)] PSN: 7530-01-000-9931 PRIVACY NOTICE: See our privacy policy on www.usps.com

PS Form **3526**, July 2014 (Page 3 of 4) PRIVACY NOTICE: See our privacy policy on www.usps.com

Moving?

Make sure your subscription moves with you!

To notify us of your new address, find your **Clinics Account Number** (located on your mailing label above your name), and contact customer service at:

Email: journalscustomerservice-usa@elsevier.com

800-654-2452 (subscribers in the U.S. & Canada)
314-447-8871 (subscribers outside of the U.S. & Canada)

Fax number: 314-447-8029

Elsevier Health Sciences Division
Subscription Customer Service
3251 Riverport Lane
Maryland Heights, MO 63043

*To ensure uninterrupted delivery of your subscription, please notify us at least 4 weeks in advance of move.

Printed and bound by CPI Group (UK) Ltd, Croydon, CR0 4YY

07/10/2024

01040504-0018